Teach Me Language

A language manual for children with autism, Asperger's syndrome and related developmental disorders.

Sabrina Freeman, Ph.D.

Lorelei Dake, B.A.

Foreword by: Shelley Davis, M.A., J.D.

Although this book is intended for parents of children with autism, Asperger's syndrome or related developmental disorders, the authors and publisher must emphasize that the exercise examples in this book are a guide to be used as part of a therapy program overseen by professional consultants, and should not be used without the professional guidance of either a behavioral consultant or speech pathologist.

Any errors and omissions are the responsibility of the first author, Dr. Sabrina Freeman.

Library of Congress Cataloging-in-Publication Data
Freeman, Sabrina
Teach me language

Includes index.
1. Autistic children--Education--Language arts.
2. Developmentally disabled children--Education--Language arts.
I. Dake, Lorelei II. Title.
LC4717.U43 1996   371.92'8046   C96-910537-1

SKF Books,
20641 46th Avenue,
Langley, B.C.
CANADA V3A 3H8

ISBN: 0-9657565-0-5
Printed in the United States of America
Second Edition

Contents

Chapter 3: General Knowledge

Chapter 4: Grammar and Syntax

Chapter 5: Advanced Language Development

Chapter 6: Academics/Language Based Concepts

Chapter 7: Therapy Schedules

Foreword by Shelley Davis, M.A., J.D.

For the majority of the fifteen years I have been working in, and later, developing and supervising behaviorally based home programs for children with autism spectrum disorders, I have been at a loss for how to answer the question, "What do we do when we finish the programs in the 'Me' book" (Teaching developmentally delayed children: The Me Book by O. Ivar Lovaas)? Finally, I can direct people to a book which provides competent guidance.

In addition to studying the programs detailed in this book, I have had the opportunity to apply many of them while working with Dr. Freeman's daughter, and later with a variety of other children. These programs have been carefully developed to strengthen areas of deficit which are often idiosyncratic to children with autism. Unfortunately, talented professionals experienced in working with high functioning autistic children are few and far between. Individuals lacking this kind of specific experience may not understand how to teach these children the complex skills delineated here, or may not fully realize the amount of repetition these children need before they can actually use certain language skills. With this book, skilled professionals can take a child that much further. Even so, a word of caution is warranted. Anyone working with children with autism, parents and professionals alike, must regularly seek the advice and consultation of someone experienced in both child development and autism - someone who can tell you "when" it's time to teach these skills. Locate someone you trust who can answer most of your questions, but who isn't afraid to say, "I don't know, let's find out together", every now and then.

The ability to ask cogent questions, and to keep asking until the answer is understood, is one of Dr. Freeman's unique gifts. In the four and a half years that I have worked with and loved Dr. Freeman's daughter, I have never tried to teach her anything that wasn't clearly explained and understood. This clarity and depth of perception is reflected in this book. No where else have I seen "why teach this skill" on each and every page. It has always surprised me that no one before this has taken the time to include this many "whys." Working with these children is simply too important to undertake it without fully understanding why we do what we do.

Good luck to all who teach and love these children. Keep on fighting the good fight.

Shelley Davis, M.A., J.D.
Behavioral Consultant
LEAP (Language and Education Assistance for Preschoolers)

1 Introduction

Fundamentals
- Why We Wrote This Book
- Who We Wrote This Book For
- Child Led vs. Therapist Led Therapy
- Understanding How to Do the Exercises
- Repetition
- Teaching Language Using a Child's Strengths
- Prompting and Fading

Commonly Asked Questions
- At What Level Does My Child Have to Be?
- Should I Teach My Child to Read?
- How Do I Get My Child to Be Table Ready?
- Will This Help My Child Be Mainstreamed?
- Why Does a Language Book Emphasize General Knowledge?
- What If My Child Knows Much of the Information Taught?
- What Does Auditory Processing Have to Do with Hearing?
- What Skills Do I Need As a Parent to Do This Therapy?
- How Often Do We Do These Drills?
- What Does This Method Achieve?
- Should I Read This Book from Cover to Cover?
- Why Are the Exercise Sheets Already Completed with Examples?
- Can I Use the "Scripts" and "Cards" Straight from the Book?

How Do I Use This Book?
- Chapter One
- Chapter Two
- Chapter Three
- Chapter Four
- Chapter Five
- Chapter Six
- Chapter Seven

Icon Definitions

Fundamentals

Why We Wrote This Book

Teach Me Language was written because we saw the need for a book to provide specific language activities designed for children with autism, Asperger's syndrome, and other related pervasive developmental disorders. There are many books advocating one therapy method over another, as well as books chronicling a child's unexpected recovery from autism. A few of these books provide information on setting up therapy in the home; however, no books that we could find give hands-on, explicit instructions for working on the language needs specific to these children, despite the fact that delayed language is one of the most common and limiting symptoms of children with developmental disorders. This book is designed to do just that. Teach Me Language introduces exercises and drills which attack language weaknesses common to children with pervasive developmental disorders.

The activities in this book were developed over a number of years through working on language difficulties amongst children with pervasive developmental disorders. These instruments are **not** intended to be put in any developmental sequence per se. Although there are language deficits common to most children with pervasive developmental disorders, every child is unique and will have strengths and weaknesses specific to that child; therefore, this book is organized topically. We have provided exercises developed to facilitate advanced language training and basic knowledge development.

Who We Wrote This Book For

Teach Me Language is designed to be used by parents, speech therapists and/or trainers as part of a therapy program where language difficulties are being addressed. There are several conditions which must be met in order for this book to be useful:

☑ The child must be a visual learner.
Children who have autism or have autistic-like disorders (i.e. pervasive developmental delays (P.D.D.) or Asperger's syndrome) are almost always visual learners. By this we mean that they are able to assimilate information when it is presented to them visually as opposed to orally. The entire book is based on this principle.

☑ The child must be table ready and relatively compliant.
One of the major challenges with this population of children is that often it is difficult to get the child to sit down at a table, even for a moment. For the parent who is beginning down the long road of therapy, getting the child table ready is step one. By table ready, we mean that the child is attentive and able to follow simple directions. The instruments

in this book will be helpful once the child is table ready. To train the child to be able to sit willingly at a table and work on language skills such as these, we strongly recommend behavioral programs to bring the child to this point. The authors can recommend Lovaas and Lovaas type training because children who have been trained this way have good table skills and have been given the building blocks to assimilate information taught to them visually. However, <u>any</u> behavioral program that brings the child to the point where s/he is table ready is needed before attempting the drills and exercises set out in the following pages. Once the child is table ready (even if only for 5 minutes at a time) then the language therapy can begin.

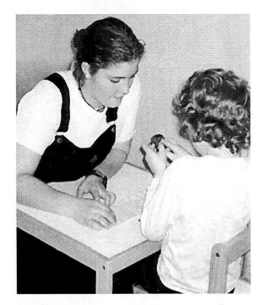

☑   The child must be able to communicate in some way.
In order to use these drills, the child must have some way to respond. If the child is verbal (even if s/he only repeats what others say - is echolalic) then eventually the child should be able to respond verbally. If the child is nonverbal, these drills can be effective if the child uses a picture communication system, a computer, or sign language, and can use one of these communication systems quite well.

Child Led versus Therapist Led Therapy

Compliance is a problem with this population of children, particularly when they are required to work on areas of weakness. The exercises in this book are most effective if the child understands that the therapist is in charge and sets the agenda. This is important because if the child is given the option to stop working whenever s/he pleases, the language drills will never be completed. It is important that the daily schedule be completed; otherwise, the child's skills will improve very slowly. To ensure that the exercises are completed, the therapist should 1) praise the child for each correct answer, 2) give the child choices where possible since the child may be more compliant if s/he has the occasional choice, and 3) reward the child upon completion of the schedule (see the section on table readiness for more information).

The language therapy is generally conducted using a written schedule. Not only does this focus the child, it also clarifies the agenda, and the goals of the session. In addition, the schedule shows the child that there is an end to the therapy session, which gives him/her a feeling of control. A typical written schedule contains a list of activities which the child checks off after each exercise completion. If placing stickers next to each activity or drawing a happy face next to the completed item is reinforcing, then the therapist should adopt this procedure. It is important to have the child "invested" in completing the daily schedule. Chapter 7 gives samples of a variety of therapy schedules, one for the child to complete, the rest for the adults to use.

Understanding How to Do the Exercises

To make this book clear for everyone, it has been written in a casual, conversational style. We try to avoid professional jargon as much as possible. The instructions for each exercise are written so that a nonprofessional can follow the technique. Every exercise is accompanied with instructions and reasons why the exercise is important to do. It is important for the parent or therapist to remember that the exercises are not self explanatory for the child. They must be introduced to the child by the adult presenting each part of the exercise, giving examples and modeling correct sample answers to the child. In order for the child to complete the exercise independently (when indicated), the child should be very familiar with the exercise, having completed the exercise many times while working with an adult.

Repetition

Each exercise provided is designed to be used over and over again using different examples within the same structure. Once the child understands the concept (by doing the exercise with new easy ideas each day), then the exercise can be made slightly more difficult. In general, only one example of each exercise is given in this book; however, these exercises should be done many times (until the child understands the concept). If the child does not understand the concept after much repetition, then an easier drill on the same concept should be introduced and/or the drill should be revised or revisited again in the future when the child is ready. Since the exercises are designed to be used many times, it is important that the therapist and/or parents be aware of the topics and answers the child likes to use or has used in the past. These children tend to give the same correct answer to the same question over and over again because they have been reinforced for that answer. The adult working with the child must encourage the use of many different (correct) answers.

Teaching Language Using a Child's Strengths

Normally-developing children learn to speak and understand the speech of others by listening; however, most children with pervasive developmental disorders do not learn well through their auditory channel. The techniques and activities described in this book attempt to teach these language delayed children about language using their visual abilities. Through strong visual channels the children can be taught oral language. In other words, once a child can 1) read a sentence, 2) understand that sentence through the visual representation, and 3) identify that sentence when someone else reads it or says it in a conversation, the child's ability to understand oral language is strengthened. This technique, however, will not work for a child whose visual channel is weaker than the oral channel.

Prompting and Fading

When a drill is first introduced, the child will have to be prompted (helped) to give the correct answer. Over time, as the child becomes competent at doing the drills, the prompts should be faded. Eventually, the child should be able to complete most drills with <u>no</u> visual prompts and, often, with no verbal prompts. When to give and fade prompts will become clear through reading the exercises.

Commonly Asked Questions

At What Level Does My Child Have to Be?

This book should be considered a <u>continuation of therapy</u> that has already begun. The child should already have a small receptive and/or expressive vocabulary. In short, the child should already know a few (5 to 10) animals, basic shapes, and basic colors. S/he should be familiar with the numbers 1 to 10, and recognize the alphabet. It is a major advantage if the child knows how to read (or decode letters). <u>Teach Me Language</u> is designed for the child who has already learned the basics of low level language. By this we mean that the child can answer questions with one word responses (or point to picture symbols to answer a question). The child should already know how to identify objects in a picture book and be able to answer simple questions such as "What is the boy doing?" or "Where is the boy?". In addition, s/he should have some basic vocabulary and should be able to read or comprehend the simple sentence patterns of noun - verb - noun such as, "The girl hit the ball", and noun-verb-prepositional phrases like, "The bird flew over the tree".

<u>Teach Me Language</u> is designed to be the next step. The drills take the child from one and two word sentences to more complex sentences and lay the foundation for conversation. The activities introduced in this book are useful for children with language delays from age five and up. The teenager with a developmental and/or language delay can also benefit from these drills as long as the exercises are adapted to be at an appropriate cognitive level i.e. the materials become more difficult yet the activities remain structured in the same way.

Should I Teach My Child to Read?

Children with pervasive developmental disorders often learn to identify letters and numbers easily. Many of them have a good memory for shapes and words and can learn to sight read. In fact, "reading" (actually decoding) is often much easier for children with autism and other pervasive developmental disorders than for their normally developing peers. For these children, reading is a significant benefit because it is a valuable prompt for speaking. Although children with developmental disorders often learn to decode at an early age, they usually do not comprehend what they are reading. The therapy technique we present in this book helps teach children to comprehend what they read at the same time as they learn to use their visual memory to help them speak and understand the spoken word. Therefore, teaching the child to read should be a high priority. We believe that it IS developmentally appropriate for these children to learn to read if reading is used as a language therapy aide and the child seems ready.

Those children who are pre-readers can still benefit from these language drills; however, they must rely on a combination of their memory and picture cards (which is less efficient). The drills are still done in much the same way for pre-readers. Many children do learn to sight read as the drills are taught to them; however, children will progress faster when they learn to decode letters. Reading can be taught using any method that has been successful with the child thus far. For example, those parents who have a Lovaas-based program can adapt the discrete trail training method to teaching phonics (outlined in the "ME" book). If the child has learned basic concepts using traditional off the shelf methods, then these methods can be used to teach phonics. There are a large variety of "How To Teach Your Child To Read" books in educational book stores. Any technique that uses basic phonics rather than just sight words is acceptable.

How Do I Get My Child to Be Table Ready?

There are many techniques available to teach the child to be table ready. The most popular techniques are based on behavioral principles. These language drills are adaptable to almost any therapy as long as the child is table ready. The bibliography below is designed to give more information regarding the behavioral method as a service to any parent whose child is not yet ready for this book; however, this book is designed for any child with language delays who is table ready, **regardless of method** used to create table readiness. *We cannot over emphasize that if the child is not yet table ready, the use of this book is premature and will not help the child.*

One well known technique is the behavioral intervention method pioneered by Ivar Lovaas at the University of California at Los Angeles (U.C.L.A.). Behavior Intervention For Children With Autism, and The Me Book, listed below, are where the parent or professional can learn to teach a child and is highly recommended:

Maurice, Catherine, 1996. Behavior Intervention For Children with Autism, Pro-Ed, Inc., 8700 Shoal Creek Boulevard, Austin, Texas 78758. Telephone: (512) 451-3246.

Lovaas, O. Ivar., 1981. Teaching Developmentally Disabled Children: The Me Book, Pro-Ed, Inc., 8700 Shoal Creek Boulevard, Austin, Texas 78758. Telephone: (512) 451-3246.

For the parent who would like to read more about the topic of language acquisition from a behavioral perspective, we include sources for additional reading:

A BIBLIOGRAPHY OF LANGUAGE ACQUISITION AND BEHAVIORAL PROGRAMS FOR CHILDREN WITH PERVASIVE DEVELOPMENTAL DISORDERS INCLUDING AUTISM

Baltaxe, C. A. M., and Simmons, J. Q. III. "Language in childhood psychosis: A review", Journal of Speech and Hearing Disorders, 1975, 40, 439-458.

Koegel, R. L., Egel, A. L., and Rincover, A. Educating and Understanding Autistic Children. San Diego: College-Hill Press, 1981.

Krantz, P. J., Zalenski, S., Hall, L. J., Fenske, E. C., and McClannahan, L. E. "Teaching complex language to autistic children", Analysis and Intervention in Developmental Disabilities. 1981,1, 259-297.

Lovaas, O. I., "Behavioral treatment and normal educational and intellectual functioning in young autistic children", Journal of Clinical and Consulting Psychology, 1987, 55, 3-9.

Lovaas, O. I. The Autistic Child: Language Development Through Behavior Modification. New York: Irvington, 1977.

Lovaas, O. I., and Smith, T. "Intensive behavioral treatment for young autistic children", In B. B. Lahey and A. E. Kazdin (Eds.), Advances in Clinical Child Psychology. (Vol. II). New York: Plenum Press, 1988. Pp. 285-324.

Schreibman, L., and Koegel, R. L "A guideline for planning behavior modification programs for autistic children", In S. M. Turner, K. S. Calhoun, and H. E. Adams (Eds.), Handbook of Clinical Behavior Therapy. Wiley-Interscience, 1981.

Will This Help My Child Be Mainstreamed?

The decision to mainstream a child is a very personal one. The language techniques taught in the book, although useful for children in both special education and regular education classrooms, are particularly important for children who are mainstreamed. In this book we provide language exercises to facilitate mainstreaming with an emphasis on the child's visual competence. Visual competence is important for the child with a pervasive developmental disorder in a mainstream, elementary environment. The child must be taught to rely on written instructions (such as those on work sheets) while the rest of the children will primarily understand directions orally. In addition, improving listening skills by relying on a visual prompt should help the child succeed in a mainstream environment where most group instruction is oral. Visual prompts are an important tool that, in some case, can be gradually faded out. In this book, there are many suggestions designed to help a child cope and succeed in school, even though much of the school day is made up of spoken language and instructions.

Why Does a Language Book Emphasize General Knowledge?

Many people are surprised that bright children with language delays do not pick up low level information (such as basic words or concepts). However, when one thinks about how much is learned through listening by small children from their environment, it is no wonder that children with developmental disorders miss much of what is seemingly mundane information. These children do not process a large amount of information that is directed toward them orally. These language delayed children may have very good memories and a fascination with minute detail due to their visual strength; however, their ability to discern the main idea from the many details may be underdeveloped. Therefore, low level general knowledge must be taught since general knowledge is the basis upon which children learn higher level information. For this reason, the book includes an important chapter on general knowledge. We suggest the child learn a structured way to gain general knowledge to be better able to identify relevant pieces of information in the environment and acquire general knowledge more naturally. In addition, the child will be more likely to pick up general auditory information from the environment. Some children will always require that information be presented visually. However, other children will begin to acquire knowledge through listening. The goal of teaching general knowledge is to strengthen the child's knowledge base and improve the child's skills to interpret general knowledge that is available naturally in the environment.

What If My Child Knows Much of the Information Being Taught?

This book is not designed for the reader to present the exercises incrementally. Furthermore, it is important not to bore a child with a concept that s/he has clearly mastered. Using the structure that is laid out in the drill, however, will enable the therapist to add components to each drill and thereby bring the drill up to the child's level. In addition, the introduction of concepts that the child may understand can help identify "holes" in the child's knowledge base. If the child is working at a level that is comparable to his/her peers, then there is no reason to work on a skill where there is no deficit. It is, however, important that the child learn the structure of the drills that are designed to teach general knowledge so that higher level information can be learned using the same structure.

What Does Auditory Processing Have to Do With Hearing?

Many parents are perplexed that their child has excellent hearing, can sing on key and imitate accents, yet cannot communicate verbally. Excellent hearing does not preclude an auditory processing problem. The technique described here uses visual prompts as well as oral prompts to help the child since information conveyed orally is more difficult for children with developmental disorders to understand. Similar to deaf children who are not taught language orally but, rather, depend on their eyesight to read lips or learn sign language, these language delayed children also learn better visually. The difference between these two groups is that children with intact hearing can use visual prompts that are eventually removed to improve and compensate for the auditory processing deficit. Once a child can read out loud (verbalizing the word), the child can eventually learn to answer in full sentences. The therapist may need to gradually remove the visual prompt, phrase by phrase, or word by word, if necessary. It is IMPERATIVE to work on the deficit, which is *auditory* understanding, while at the same time relying on the strength, which is *visual* processing.

Many of the ideas in this book use the child's visual strength as a crutch which is slowly faded out so the child comes to rely solely on auditory processing. An example of this is an advanced activity to teach the child to take notes (designed for a child in 3rd grade or higher). At first, the therapist shows the child how to take notes from an easy written sentence. Then, the therapist reads a sentence that the child is very familiar with. The child takes notes as the therapist reads. Once the child understands the concept of note-taking, the therapist reads an easy unfamiliar sentence and the child takes notes, with prompting from the therapist. Eventually, the child is introduced to taking notes from easy paragraphs by listening to the therapist read. This is an example of a skill that is learned over a number of months in which the initial exercise relies on a visual prompt that is eventually faded.

As a Parent, What Skills Do I Need to Do This?

This book has been organized so that parents with minimal experience can do the language activities and drills with the child without specialized training. Parents or paraprofessionals who have organized or been involved in intensive behavioral programs will find these drills and activities easy to do. Those parents who have watched effective speech pathologists work with their children should also have little difficulty implementing the ideas in this book. The activities are designed for easy use. Before every drill, there is a HOW TO section that must be read prior to engaging the child in the drill. In addition, where appropriate, there is a PROBLEM section which attempts to anticipate common problems. These two sections must be read by everyone prior to doing a drill. The last section, the WHY section, is an explanation of why the drill needs to be done with the child. The WHY sections in the book are intended as further information for the curious parent or therapist, but are not required to implement the drills.

How Often Do We Do These Drills?

This question is an important one. Very often children do not progress very quickly in language therapy because it is assumed that working on drills once a week is sufficient. This is an unfortunate and incorrect assumption. If one wants to see quick progress, drills must be done ONCE A DAY. Certain drills must be done several times a day. To illustrate, one activity asks the child to tell the parent about what the child did at school. In order for some children to understand what is required of them, this drill may have to be done four times a day. At school, either the teacher or aide should ask the child to name four things s/he did at school. Then when the child arrives home, one parent should ask the child what s/he did at school today. When the other parent comes home, the child should then be asked by the other parent what s/he did at school today. Finally, the child should be asked by a sibling or therapist what s/he did at school today. After a couple of weeks, the child will probably be able to recall four things s/he did at school that day. If this particular drill is not done intensively, it may take the child months to understand what s/he is being asked to talk about.

What Does This Method Achieve?

The technique we present here is designed to improve communication with the child through the child's strongest channel which is visual. In addition, this method teaches the child to use visual cues such as pictures or words as prompts. If the child has the ability to form words (often these children repeat words or phrases at first -- are echolalic), then the method exercises their oral, expressive ability as well as receptive skills. By introducing language visually, the child develops the skills to understand the structure of language in much the same way as an adult learns a foreign language. The visual language can then be used as a prompt for the expressive language. Through all drills, the therapist or parent gives verbal directions to the child while using a visual cue. The child eventually understands those directions without a visual prompt and is more likely to understand other adults when they give similar directions. *The basic premise is that patterned language gives the child tools to understand, internalize, and recall basic information.*

Should I Read This Book from Cover to Cover?

No. The parent or therapist should first go to Chapter 7 and look at the suggested schedule of activities to start out with. Then the pages relevant to the particular drill that is to be taught should be read and the materials assembled (if necessary). In order to set up a customized therapy schedule, the parent or therapist should skim each chapter and read the drills that are 1) at the child's level, and 2) address the child's deficits.

Why Are the Exercise Sheets Already Completed with Examples?

In order for everyone to understand how to perform the drills, the book includes actual facsimiles of the drill sheets, filled out as examples of how the drills are done. In this way, the "How To" section is demonstrated with a completed drill. A set of empty exercise sheets will be available separately by Fall 1996.

Can I Use the "Scripts" and "Cards" Straight Out of the Book?

The scripts need to be presented to the child in a much larger format than is possible to put in the book. Therefore, we suggest that the script be enlarged using a photocopier or written neatly on a blackboard or large piece of paper. The cards can be photocopied straight out of the book and used. Card stock or laminating paper is a good idea since some of the cards will be heavily used.

How Do I Use This Book?

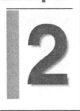

Chapter 1

This chapter introduces the book. It tells the parent whether their child will benefit from the book and answers commonly asked questions about the level the child must be at to benefit. In addition, the way the parent or therapist should use the activities and drills in the book is explained.

Chapter 2

Chapter 2 provides activities to improve social language. The emphasis is to improve the child's ability to speak about a single topic, as well as to converse with a peer. There are drill sheets that teach appropriate social questions and answers, and teach emotions. Most importantly, we introduce drills to teach the child critical thinking skills such as how to discern "Safe" from "Dangerous" and "Problems" from "Non-problems" while improving his/her ability to understand and use language.

Chapter 3

This chapter includes exercises designed to train the child to pick up general information. We introduce 1) activities and materials on many different topics and 2) drills designed to increase comprehension of factual knowledge. In addition, the child is taught to compare and contrast, to define vocabulary, and to use true/false concepts based on general information the child learns.

Chapter 4

The fourth chapter concentrates on grammar and syntax. In this chapter, the child is given different opportunities to learn the structure of language. Several language games and activities designed to concentrate on particular parts of language are introduced with the hope that once the child understands and uses the structure of the language, s/he will be able to create or assemble original sentences.

Chapter 5

Chapter Five concentrates on increasing the child's functional knowledge and written expression of that knowledge. In this chapter, we introduce structured paragraph, story, and letter writing. In addition, we offer drills designed to improve the child's ability to recall and communicate personal, daily experiences.

Chapter
6

Chapter 6 is designed to work on language based academic concepts. In this chapter, we provide fiction based comprehension exercises and several activities designed to reinforce that comprehension skill. In addition, drills to address math <u>word</u> problems, dictionary skills, increasing vocabulary, and sequencing with money, time, calendar and numbers are introduced. Finally, the chapter explains how to teach the child to take written notes from auditory information.

Chapter
7

Chapter 7 presents several therapy schedules and gives the parent or therapist an idea of how to set up a daily schedule, specifying the type of exercises to do depending upon the child's level.

Icons and Type Styles In This Book

Teach Me Language has many sections with a variety of instruments and exercises. In order to make it easy for the reader to make sense of the organization, we have used symbols in the margins to denote the type of section on each page.

HOW TO
Everywhere a key symbol is used, the text is explaining HOW TO use or do something.

WHY
The symbol used when the text is explaining WHY is represented by the question mark . These first two symbols are generally on the page which introduces the section.

EXERCISE/DRILL
The exercise book symbol represents an exercise or drill sheet. The sheets in the book have all been filled out to illustrate what the completed drill looks like. Empty sheets may be purchased separately.

SCRIPTS
The scroll represents the various scripts we include in the book. The scripts are to be read with the child many times, over several therapy sessions. The scripts are designed to introduce the child to concepts in a general way before s/he does the work sheet relating to the concept being taught.

SAMPLES
Throughout the book, samples of paragraphs and lists are given. These samples can be used to begin therapy. When they have been exhausted, the parent or therapist can easily create more samples following the same format.

MATERIALS/CARDS
This symbol is used when materials or cards need to be photocopied and cut out for use in therapy. All the cards are reproducible on a photocopier.

LANGUAGE GAMES
The jester icon is used to indicate a language exercise conducted in the form of a game.

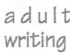

ADULT HANDWRITING
Throughout the book, whenever the therapist is supposed to prepare a "work" sheet or write down answers the child gives, we indicate this on the sample drill sheets with an adult writing style in grey.

CHILD HANDWRITING
When the child is required to complete the exercise by themselves, we indicate this on the sample drill sheets with a child's writing style in grey.

2 Social Language

What We Mean By Social Language
Simple Word Associations
- Exercises

Building Analogies
- Exercises

Topical Conversation
- Exercises and Scripts

Finding Out About Someone
- Games and Exercises

Verbal Reciprocal Comments
- Exercises

Joint Attention
- Exercises

Contingent Statements
- Exercises and Materials

Conversation
- Exercises, Scripts, and Games

Emotions
- Exercises and Scripts

Critical Thinking
- Deciding Who To Listen To - Exercises and Scripts
- Safe and Dangerous - Exercises and Scripts
- Problems and Solutions - Exercises and Scripts
- Being Made Fun Of - Exercises and Scripts

Daily Language Requirements
- Ordering Food
- Answering the Telephone

Fact or Opinion
- Exercises and Materials

What Do We Mean By Social Language?

In this chapter, we concentrate on activities designed to promote social language. By social language we refer to the daily banter that goes on between children to facilitate social interaction. Each drill is designed to attack the problem of spontaneous speech from a different angle. The drills at the beginning of the chapter (such as simple word associations, contingent words, pretend play, building analogies, easy topical conversation, finding out about someone, and joint attention) are generally easier than those near the end of the chapter, although they do not have to be done strictly in the order presented. It is important to begin with drills that the child is certain to master. The parent or therapist should not assume that the child can master the more difficult exercises before doing the easier exercises.

Drills to address emotions are also provided, since this area is often a problem for children with autism. The basic emotions (happy, sad, mad, scared, proud, frustrated, and worried) are covered here. As the child grows, emotions become more complex and, therefore, more complex scripts will be required. The basic format of the emotion scripts provided in this chapter can be used to create more complex emotion scripts. Advanced emotion scripts contain complex situations which are used to bring across the subtleties of emotions which are abstract in nature (e.g. envy, hurt feelings, insult, worry).

Chapter 2 also covers critical thinking, since this is a difficult subject for children with developmental disorders typically must be taught to think critically. The critical thinking drills cover subjects important to the child's well-being such as "Deciding Who to Listen To", "Deciding What to Do", "Safe and Dangerous", "Problems and Solutions", "Being Made Fun Of", and "Being Hurt". We **strongly** encourage the parent or therapist to customize any or all scripts and create new scripts to accommodate their particular child's needs. The examples used must be relevant to each child. We have also included drills to concentrate on the child's recall of his/her day as well as practical language-rich situations such as answering the telephone or ordering a meal. We also introduce advanced drills in the section on Fact vs. Opinion. Finally, several games have been included to promote communication.

How To Teach Simple Word Associations

Prerequisite: Before introducing this drill, the child must be able to match things that go together e.g. a shoe and a sock.

There are two ways to teach this drill.

1. The therapist writes down two word pairs. First the focus should be on nouns and adjectives (adjective-noun e.g. green frog). Here is an example of the way a therapist would introduce the drill.

Therapist: "John, green - frog" (reading the word pairs). Why do these words go together?"

The therapist can prompt verbally or in writing if necessary at first.

Therapist: "because a _____ is _____".

Once the child understands how to use "is", then the therapist should gradually introduce other linking verbs such as *tastes, sounds, feels,* etc. At first, the therapist's goal is to have the child begin to verbalize the reason that the word pair goes together on his/her own, regardless of the linking verb used.

2. Another way to do this drill is by writing down a word (a noun) and introducing the drill as follows.

Therapist: "John, what goes with (a) _____."

The therapist should write down what the child says, and then ask: "why do _____ and _____ go together?"

The therapist should prompt the child to say "because a _____ is _____." It is fine for the child to give a different noun or verb than what the therapist has thought of, as long as the child has a valid reason for putting the words together. These children often generate associations that are not considered typical. These associations are valid, however, if the child can supply an appropriate reason. The therapist may have to prompt the reason or response in a different form (e.g. pencil-paper, "because a pencil writes <u>on</u> paper").

Eventually, the child should be able to describe why two words go together verbally only when presented with paired words without the visual prompt.

 # Why Do This Drill?

The purpose of this drill is to get the child to 1) see and verbalize the relationship between words, 2) develop the ability to answer Why questions, and 3) understand the concept of Why - Because. In addition, word associations help auditory comprehension in daily life. For example, if the child is asked to "Go get a pencil and paper", s/he will be able to easily carry out this instruction because it makes sense to the child. Ability to associate words also leads to the association of events with details e.g. a birthday party is associated with a cake, presents, balloons, etc.

Simple Word Associations

The simple word association exercise can be done in two ways. The way to introduce this drill is to have the therapist write down a word pair and ask the child why the two words go together. The second way to do this drill is to have the child give a word that relates to the one word the therapist suggests. Then the child must "explain" why s/he chose the word (e.g. why s/he chose flower to go with butterfly). Once the child can do this with relative ease, s/he can move on to "The Contingent Word" exercise.

Simple Word Associations

Word Paired Word	Reason
butterfly - flower	Because a butterfly sits on a flower.
swim - water	Because we swim in the water.
yellow - crayon	Because a crayon is yellow.
monkey - banana	Because a monkey eats a banana.
blanket - bed	Because a blanket is on the bed.

How To Teach Contingent Words

Contingent words in work much the same way as do word associations. The therapist begins by saying a word, and then writing down that word. Then the child must say any word that is remotely related to the first word. The therapist makes a word association based on the child's word, and the child makes a word association based on the therapist's new word. This turn taking should be done with the entire sheet. If the child has trouble completing this exercise, then the therapist should break down the exercise line by line instead of completing the entire sheet. Some children will pick this drill up immediately; others will take longer to grasp the drill. The therapist can help the child by starting off with subjects that the child likes and by using examples the child understands. For example, if the therapist starts by writing **Disneyland**, then the child should be prompted to say anything that is related to Disneyland. The therapist must take the child's suggestion, and find another topic which is unrelated to Disneyland, but related to the child's suggestion. For example, the drill might resemble the following pattern. Therapist: "Disneyland"; Child: "Mickey Mouse"; Therapist: "black ears"; Child: "feet"; Therapist: "shoes"; Child: "pants"; Therapist: "dress"; Child: "doll"; Therapist: "Barbie"; Child: "toy", and so on. This drill is usually quite enjoyable for the child because s/he can communicate without having to put thought in an entire sentence. This exercise can be used for years since each time it is done, the word associations are different.

Note: It is important that the child not be allowed to continue with the same train of thought over many turns. The idea is for the child to listen to the last word, and come up with an association for that one word (and not previous words or ideas).

Variation: A good variation to this drill was developed by Shelley Davis, a very talented behavioral consultant who heads many programs for children with pervasive developmental disorders. Once Ms. Davis completes the above drill, she asks the child, "Why do (word) and (word) go together?" She then prompts the child to say, "Because (word) and (word) are both (word)" or "Because (word) goes with (word)". After a while, the child is able to explain the relationship between the two words and has grasped the "Why-Because" relationship.

Why Teach Contingent Words?

Contingent words give the child an opportunity to express his/her thoughts without having to frame them in a full sentence. This gives the therapist an opportunity to see how much the child knows when the child is not bogged down with grammatical structure. In addition, the Contingent Word drill shows the therapist the child's areas of weakness in terms of gaps in general knowledge. This drill is also a good way to work on both simple and complex adjectives (colors and shapes, and emotions) and opposites.

Contingent Word Work Sheet

This exercise structures a conversation of sorts, since the child is able to share his/her thoughts without putting them into a sentence. There is turn taking where the child and the therapist both must concentrate on what the other is saying, since the next word must relate to the preceding word. Once the sheet is completed, the child can choose one of the lines and explain why the two words go together. This exercise is one of the easiest exercises with which to start the social language chapter.

Contingent Words

rain — wet — water — swimming — summer

beach — sand — ocean — grey — kitten

soft — loud — siren — fire — hot

sun — sky — moon — night — stars

because Saturn is bright
because Saturn has rings
because we wear a ring on our finger
because a finger has a nail

bright — Saturn — rings — finger — nail

How To Teach Analogy Building

The therapist should begin by slowly describing the completed sheet. She should go through the entire sheet, pointing out groups of two words that relate to each other. Once she has completed the sheet, then she should present the child with a new activity sheet and have the child create the two word relationships. If the child has difficulty with this, the therapist should heavily prompt the child until s/he understands the structure of the drill. If the child has a very difficult time with this drill, the therapist should create an entire sheet of two word pairs which all have the same relationship. Once the child understands the pattern, s/he will be able to complete the drill.

This drill lends itself to an infinite number of analogies, each with a different skill level required. The example uses objects and their colors which is very easy; however, the analogies can be made much more difficult. Examples include animals and their classifications, objects and their functions, countries and their continents.

Why Teach Building Analogies?

Analogy building develops the child's critical thinking skills as well as an understanding of the relationship between different parts of language. For example, nouns have descriptive properties, verbs have functions, and adjectives describe nouns. In addition, through analogy building, the child is required to create a full sentence to describe the relationship of these two concepts. Furthermore, the relationship between the words is made explicit through the use of phrases like, "is the color of"; "is the type of"; "is a country in"; "is a planet in" and so on.

Building Analogies (Identifying Word Relationships)

This exercise builds the child's critical thinking skills. The therapist should do several word pairs before having the child come up with these words on his/her own. In addition, the therapist should go through a completed sheet with the child before requiring the child to do this on his/her own. Once the child understands the relationship that the therapist would like him/her to create, then the child should try the sheet on his own coming up with different relationship sentences.

Building Analogies (Identifying Word Relationships)

In each box an arrow is drawn from one word to another. On the line below, tell how or why the words go together (write a relationship sentence). Then find 2 other words that go together in the same way. Write the relationship sentence for the 2 words you choose. Then think of 2 more words that could go together in the same way and write your own relationship sentence.

Contingent Words

grass   banana

dirt   green

yellow   brown

Relationship Sentence: _____Yellow is the color of a banana._____

_____

Relationship Sentence: _____Green is the color of grass._____

_____

2 more words that go together in the same way: _Red - Strawberry_

Relationship Sentence: _Red is the color of strawberries._

_____

How To Teach Pretend Play

The therapist selects several different, unrelated, non-play objects. Good examples are a spoon, a cup and a straw. These items must be objects the child knows how to use or knows the function of. An illustration of how to perform this drill is below:

The first object is a spoon. The therapist holds it up and says,
Therapist: "Suzie, what can we use this for?"
Child: "Spoon".
Therapist: "Yes. This is a spoon. What can we USE this for?"
Child: "Eating."
Therapist: "Yes. We eat with a spoon." "We can PRETEND it is a guitar" (Therapist strums on the spoon as if it were a guitar).
Therapist: "What else can we use it for".
Child: "Tail?"
Therapist: "Yes, we can pretend it is a tail". The therapist helps the child pretend by guiding the child's hand with the spoon.

Problems: Some children quickly pick up on the game. Other children take a long time to understand the concept of **pretend**. For children who do not understand the drill, the therapist can model the answer for a few specific objects. The child will eventually come to understand that s/he is expected to come up with ideas that traditionally are not associated with the item.

Why Work On Pretend Play?

The purpose of this exercise is to have the child realize that things can be used for functions other than originally intended. This will improve the child's ability to problem solve, imagine and create. The exercise helps the child to think differently by looking at objects in a new light. This is an attempt to work on the process of generalizing and abstracting - two areas in which children with developmental delays often show deficits.

Pretend Play Work Sheet

Pretend play is one of the deficits typical in children with various pervasive developmental disorders. Yet, it is an important social skill since much play involves pretending amongst younger children. This activity structures pretend play in its simplest form. Once the child understands the exercise, it is a good idea to begin very simple pretend exercises with dolls. For example, the child can be taught to pretend that the doll is swimming, eating or going to sleep. Once the child understands pretend play with dolls, then the next step is to create a very simple story about a doll going to do an activity. Once the child can tell a story about a doll, it is a good idea to create scripts that can be acted out using dolls. Some children will take these skills and generalize them in their free time. This work sheet is for the therapist and should not be used by the child.

Play With Inanimate Objects

	Item	Response	Demonstrates Play
1.	cup	hat	puts on head
2.	lid	cookie	eats
3.	spoon	guitar	plays the guitar
4.	chair	house	crawls under
5.	pen	phone	talks into

Topical Conversation

SHEET 1

Using the topical conversation form provided, the therapist has the child choose something to talk about. For example, the therapist should say, "Jane, what do you want to talk about?" If the child does not choose, the therapist can give him/her a choice between 2 familiar topics. Then, the therapist must write down the topic on the line at the top of the page (preferably one word but the whole sentence if necessary). The therapist should then say, "Jane, tell me something about _____, "then, "Tell me something else about _____", etc. Prompts may be needed such as, "Tell me about the shape/size/color", etc..

The therapist must write down, in single word format, 4 things that the child says.

The therapist then has the child talk about the topic by pointing to the form and saying, "Jane, tell me about _____". The therapist should help the child use complete sentences to tell about the 4 things.

After the child describes the topic, the therapist should try to maintain the conversation through 2 more turns by asking general questions such as, "Where can we get?" or "Where can we see ___?", etc.

The following day, the therapist should repeat the drill using the same topic without the form to see whether the child can recall what s/he said on her own. The therapist should look for original statements about the topic - this is the eventual goal of the exercise.

 # Why Teach Topical Conversation?

The purpose of the topical conversation is to develop the child's ability to talk on a topic for an extended period. In addition, it is important to develop this skill on a large number of different topics so the child is not stuck with one or two conversations and people are not always stuck speaking with the child about the same topics. Examples of topics which are of interest to many children are: Disneyland; the local amusement park; Power Rangers (or other latest craze); McDonald's restaurant; Barbie's; popular computer games. It is important to remember that the goal is to have the child talk to his/her peers; therefore, the therapist must take the cue of what the latest fad is from the child's normally developing peers. Also, it is important to make sure that the topic is age-appropriate. For example, it is acceptable for a preschooler to talk about Sesame Street characters; however, a first grade child should be talking about Disney, not Sesame Street, characters.

Topical Conversation Activity Sheet (1)

This exercise teaches the child the basic structure of a conversation in which the child must describe a topic and answer questions on that topic. This is a prerequisite for conversations in which the child both asks and answers questions. The therapist should make sure the topic chosen is one which the child knows something about.

Topical Conversation Activity Sheet (1)

TOPIC:
*(what you want
to talk about)*

The Park

DETAILS:
*(the important things
you want to say about
the main idea)*

1   swings

2   slide

3   sandbox

4   bench

Topical Conversation

SHEET 2

Prerequisite: Before introducing Sheet 2, the child must be very proficient at the Sheet 1 Topical Conversation drill. The therapist should proceed as in Sheet 1, taking care to write down one word per thought (e.g. "Park" instead of "I like to go to the park"). After each point the child makes about the topic, the therapist should prompt the child to say something about that point. For example, the drill would sound something like the following:

Therapist: "What do you want to talk about?"
Child: "Park." (Therapist writes "Park").
Therapist: "Tell me something about the park."
Child: "Park has grass." (Therapist writes "grass").
Therapist: "What can you tell me about grass?"
Child: "Green."
Therapist: "Tell me something else about the park." (The therapist should point to 2. on the sheet).
Child: "Park has swings." (Therapist writes "swings").
Therapist: "Tell me about the swings."
Child: "Swings are fun." (Therapist writes "fun").

The interaction continues until the sheet is completed. Then the therapist reverbalizes the topic with the descriptors and elaborations i.e. The therapist says, "I like to go to the park. The park has grass. The grass is green. The park has swings. Swings are fun." Finally, the child is given the opportunity to reverbalize the topic using the sheet as a prompt. Once the child understands the structure of the exercise (after several times), then s/he should be asked to reverbalize the topic twice, once with the sheet, and once without the sheet.

Afterward, the therapist should try to maintain the conversation through 2 more turns by asking him/her general questions about the topic such as, "What can we do at the park?", "Where do we see a park?", etc.

Another activity that can strengthen this process is to have the child use her topical conversational outline to write a short paragraph on the topic (1 to 2 lines). This can be done on the computer if the child is good with a keyboard, or through writing if this is a stronger skill.

Why Teach Topical Conversation?

It is very important that the child be able to talk about many topics since this ability gives the child more opportunity to become involved in conversation. This exercise improves the child's conversational flow and helps him/her understand, follow and participate in conversations. The eventual goal is for the child to participate in conversation spontaneously. Topical conversation drills also help prepare a child to give information on a topic at school e.g. for show and tell, sharing, or any oral presentation.

Topical Conversation Activity Sheet (2)

This more advanced exercise is similar to the initial exercise. The difference here is that the child must elaborate on what s/he is describing. This drill teaches the child the purpose of adjectives or descriptive words in language and is a prerequisite for conversations in which the child both asks and answers questions. The therapist should make sure that the topic chosen is one which the child knows something about.

Topical Conversation Activity Sheet (2)

TOPIC:
(what you want to talk about)

Park

DETAILS:
(the important things you want to say about the main idea)

① grass

green

② swings

fun

③ field

ball

④ slide

down

How To Maintain Conversation Skills

This drill teaches the child how to start and maintain a conversation. At first, the conversation will be very structured. As time passes, the child should be encouraged to gradually leave the structured template. The Topical Conversation Activity Sheet (1), and question cue cards (which immediately follow) are used for this exercise.

The therapist starts the conversation by asking the child,
Therapist: "Ask me about my day."
Child (being prompted by the sheet): "What did you do today?"
Therapist (choosing a topic of interest to the child): "I went to the beach."
Child (using a question cue card): "What did you do?"
Therapist: "I went swimming."
Child (using a cue card): "What did you see?"
Therapist: "I saw kids making sand castles."
Child: "What did you eat?"
Therapist: "I ate a hamburger and fries."
The therapist should continue with the child until the conversation naturally concludes, generally taking 3 to 4 turns. Initially there is no conversational flow with this activity; therefore, it should be done several times as a script. Eventually, the conversation should flow and the script (or the question cue cards) should be removed. Examples of other scripts, and sheets are "Finding Out About Someone", "Movie Scripts" and "Conversational Rules". Once the child has mastered the questions from these forms, the therapist should set up a situation where the child is given the opportunity to ask non-therapists these questions.

Problems: Occasionally, a child may become rigid about the order that the questions are asked. One solution to this is to mix the order of the questions or reintroduce the questions in cue card form, shuffling the cards each time. The idea is for the child to become accustomed to the questions being asked in different order. In addition, if the child can learn to ask a number of questions in a different order, the child's speech will sound more natural than if s/he rigidly goes through the entire sequence in the same order every time.

Note: A conversation Record has been included as a way to have the child generalize his/her conversation skills. This record requires the cooperation of the teacher and/or school aide. Eventually, the child should be able to use the record on his/her own.

Why Teach Conversation Skills?

Conversations are the way people find out about their immediate world. Children with language delays do not obtain conversation skills naturally. This drill is designed to manually teach a skill that is automatic in most normally developing children. Through providing a variety of topics, the child may come to realize that these same questions can be asked in a number of different situations and that initiating conversation can be a fun thing to do.

Cards To Teach Conversation

These are reproducible cards to be used as explained on the previous page. They can be photocopied onto card stock to ensure their durability.

What did you do today?	**What did you see?**
What did you do?	**What did you eat?**
What did you drink?	**Who did you play with?**

Rules for Talking With Friends Script

The Rules for Talking With Friends Script should be read over with the child on several occasions including immediately before a child comes to play. The idea is for the child to understand the implicit rules of talking with friends by making the rules explicit. Each rule should be practiced and reinforced until the child internalizes the rules.

Rules for Talking With Friends

1. When you want to say something to someone, say their name first to get their attention.

2. Always look at the person you are talking to.

3. Face the person you are talking to or turn your body towards them.

4. Always listen to what the other person is saying.

Movie Conversation

These are reproducible cards that should be photocopied onto card stock and then used when structuring a conversation on movies. The idea is to give the child a visual prompt to start off the sentence. This structure allows him/her to express opinions about movies while teaching the vernacular the children use when talking among themselves. Eventually, the child will memorize these sentence openings and, hopefully, use them to express themselves on other related topics as well i.e. books, videos, performances.

Did you see the movie...?

Wasn't it cool when ...

What part did you like?

Remember the part about ...

I liked it when ...

The best part was when ...

Yeah,... was a pretty good movie.

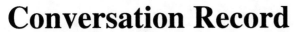

Conversation Record

The child should have a Conversation Record taped to his/her desk everyday at school and at home during therapy. If this is done consistently, the child will be engaged in conversation 6 times per day, which is the minimum requirement for the child. At first, the child will need considerable prompting until s/he realizes that s/he is accountable for initiating and recording some sort of conversation 3 times per setting. The child must learn to fill in the form (with heavy prompting at first, if necessary). After the child knows how to complete the form independently, a reinforcement/consequence system must be built in to motivate the child to complete the form. For example, if s/he engages in conversation at least 3 times, s/he receives a reward (s/he earns something special). The key to this drill's effectiveness is to motivate the child to have a conversation, and eventually fade out the form and the reward without diminishing the conversational behavior.

Conversation Record

Date: _October 10th, 1995_ Where: _at school_

		Who	What
☒	Ask a question; Say/ask 2 more things	David	game you like / Nintendo / math workshop
☒	Ask a question; Say/ask 2 more things	Joey	sport you like / soccer / baseball
☒	Ask a question; Say/ask 2 more things	Josh	do you have a dog / I like dogs / I have a frog

Finding Out About Someone

The therapist should model the questions in the "Finding Out About Someone" drill and then prompt the child to ask the question. Once the child knows the question to ask, the therapist must use the one word written on the form as a prompt. The therapist can say, "Let's find out about Suzie." The therapist should ask the child all the questions on the form and then say, "Ask me." She can prompt the child by saying, "Jane, what do you like to eat?" Once the therapist gives her answer, they can continue with the next question. The "play" question should be asked, "**Who** do you like to play with?", and the "go" question should be asked, "**Where** do you like to go?" Once the sheet is completed, the therapist should say, "Tell about what I like to do". Using the point form responses on the sheet to cue the child, s/he should talk about the therapist's preferences such as, "Jane likes to eat hamburgers." At first, this will need to be prompted but the prompts should be faded quickly.

Part of conversation is listening to answers, not just asking questions. In order to have the child practice listening to the answers s/he has asked, the therapist can have the child go into another room and ask someone a question from the sheet e.g "Go find out what Carol likes to eat." Then the child listens to the answer, and returns. The therapist then asks, "What does Carol like to eat?". The therapist then writes down the person's answer based on what the child has told the therapist.

This is a very good drill to do with a normally developing peer ONCE THE CHILD IS GOOD AT THE DRILL. In this way, the peer learns about the child's preferences, and the child is required to listen to the peer. Prior to using this drill with a peer, this is a good exercise to do with as many different adults as possible.

There are four drill sheets for this activity. Once the child masters the first sheet, the next two sheets should be relatively easy for the child to learn. The fourth sheet is meant to be customized for the child using questions the child would like to know the answer to. For example, if s/he is interested in boats, then a question asking about the person's favorite boat would be a good question. Once the child is good at asking the questions on all four sheets, then the one-word cue cards should be used. Eventually, the cards should be faded out and the child should have internalized a sufficient number of questions s/he can use to have a conversation.

Why Teach the "Finding Out" Drill?

The "Finding Out" exercise is very important to teach since children with developmental delays do not have the language to ask appropriate questions of peers. When they are interested in a peer, it is difficult for them to find the words with which to form the question. By teaching social scripts (questions that ask people about themselves), the goal is to have the child internalize these questions so s/he has the tools to be social in a verbal manner. In addition, these children will be asked the same questions by their peers. They should be familiar with these questions and any other questions that are confronted regularly (e.g. if the child is asked about their favorite Ninja Turtle, it is a good idea to teach them to choose their preference, and then be able to ask that question themselves). This drill also shows the child that s/he must listen to the response of the conversant because conversations change course based on the response of the other person.

Finding Out About Someone (1)

This exercise is designed to give the child the necessary tools to find out about another person. The first sheet includes basic questions. The child should use the sheet to ask people these questions. Once the child has mastered these questions, the next sheet should be introduced and sheet (1) should be used periodically to maintain the questions. Eventually, the sheet should be faded out and the child should be able to ask people questions from memory.

Finding Out About Someone #1

Ask __Jane__ questions about what s/he likes.

1. _____eat_____   _____hamburger_____

2. _____drink_____   _____milk shake_____

3. _____do_____   _____play baseball_____

4. _____play with_____   _____John, Sue_____

5. _____go_____   _____Disneyland_____

Finding Out About Someone (2)

This exercise is designed to give the child the necessary tools to find out about another person. This second sheet includes questions that are slightly more advanced than the first. As in the first sheet, the child should use this sheet to ask people these questions. Once the child has mastered these questions, the third sheet should be introduced and this sheet (2) should be used periodically to maintain the questions. Eventually, the sheet should be faded out and the child should be able to ask people questions from memory.

Finding Out About Someone #2

Ask ___Jane___ questions about what s/he likes.

1. _____ movie _____   Pocahontas

2. _____ book _____   Hop on Pop

3. _____ animal _____   dog

4. _____ color _____   pink

5. _____ friend _____   Stacy

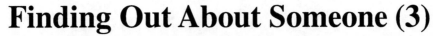

Finding Out About Someone (3)

This exercise is designed to give the child the necessary tools to find out about another person. This third sheet includes questions that are slightly more advanced than questions on the first and second sheets. As in the previous sheets, the child should use this sheet to ask people these questions. Once the child has mastered these questions, then the therapist and the child should use the fourth sheet to think of some questions that are truly interesting to the child. Eventually, all the sheets should be faded out and the child should be able to ask people questions from memory.

Finding Out About Someone #3

Ask _Jane_ questions about what s/he likes.

1. old/birthday _____ March 12, 1988

2. live _____ San Francisco

3. family _____ 3 people

4. brothers/sisters _____ 1 brother

5. pet _____ Yes

Finding Out About Someone (4)

This exercise is designed to give the child the necessary tools to find out about another person. This fourth sheet includes questions the child cares about. These questions should be of genuine interest to the child. Eventually, all the sheets should be faded out and the child should be able to ask people questions from memory. *NOTE: They can ask questions they have learned from the first three sheets but not in the same order. It is good if they can come up with new questions; however, that is an advanced skill.*

Finding Out About Someone #4

Ask ___Jane___ questions about what s/he likes.

1. __favorite instrument__   ___Piano___

2. __computer game__   ___Math Dodger___

3. __favorite restaurant__   ___McDonald's___

4. __favorite song__   ___Whistle while you work___

5. __kind of donut__   ___glazed with sprinkles___

Game Cards For Finding Out About Someone

These are reproducible game cards to be used as explained on the previous page. They can be photocopied onto card stock to ensure their durability.

color	book
eat	drink
do	play with
go	game

Game Cards For Finding Out About Someone

These are reproducible game cards to be used as explained on the previous page. They can be photocopied onto card stock to ensure their durability.

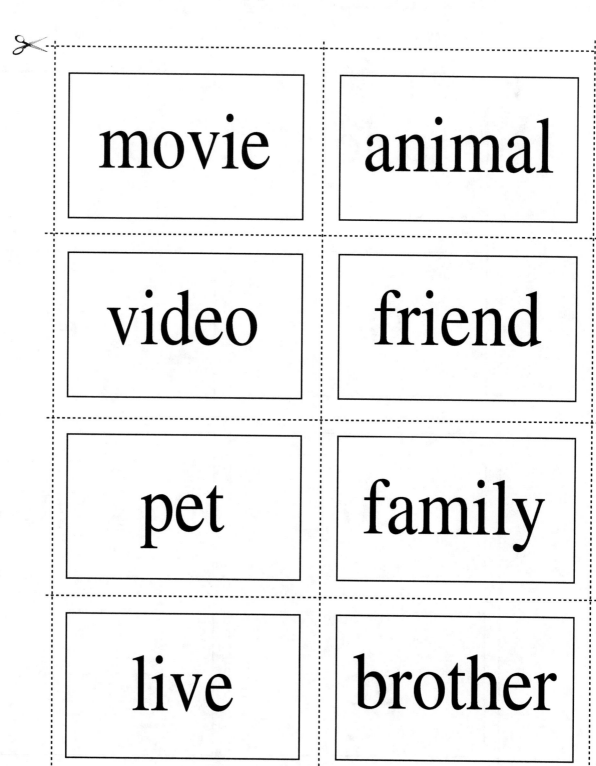

Game Cards For Finding Out About Someone

These are reproducible game cards to be used as explained on the previous page. They can be photocopied onto card stock to ensure their durability. The blank cards are designed to have the questions that interest the child included.

sister	aunt
uncle	_____
_____	_____
_____	_____

How To Teach Verbal Reciprocal Comments

The therapist begins by making a statement such as, "I like to eat pizza". Then the child is prompted to say, "I like to eat _____". Then the therapist makes another statement such as, "I like to go to the Discovery Zone", and prompts the child to say, "I like to go to _____". After a while, the therapist should not have to prompt the child to repeat the structure of what she is saying since the child will understand the pattern. The therapist should do this drill with the child until all the possible, obvious subjects have been covered and the child clearly understands the pattern and can come up with the correct matching comment.

This is the typical conversational pattern of many preschoolers. They really do not relate to what the other child is saying except to use it as a cue to talk about themselves.

Problems: If the child has difficulties with this drill, it is a good idea to use a visual cue to talk about. For example, the therapist can give the child a toy, take a toy for herself and say, "I have a car". She should then prompt the child to say, "I have a train". Then the therapist should describe one thing about her toy, and have the child describe the same thing about his/her own toy. Once the child understands this game, the reciprocal verbal comment drill can be taught.

Variations: This drill can also be done with clothing, hair/eye color etc. (Example: "I have blue pants").

Note: This is a fun exercise to do with a playmate sitting in a circle since typically developing children love to talk about themselves. When a peer is included, this drill teaches the child to listen to his/her peers and take turns.

Why Teach Reciprocal Verbal Comments?

The child must be taught verbal reciprocity since this mechanism does not work well in children with language delays. Therefore, by practicing reciprocity in drill form, the child becomes accustomed to asking, answering, and commenting. These are the tools necessary to engage in social conversation. This drill may not increase the child's social motivation; however, if and when the child does feel like joining in a conversation, s/he will have the ability if this activity is done with the child beforehand.

How To Teach Joint Attention

The Joint Attention exercise is designed to increase the child's ability to share his/her interests with another person. This drill can be done anytime, anywhere. The following are examples of how to do the drill.

At home:

The therapist should get up and have the child stand up. Then the therapist says, "Show me some things around your house/in your room etc... Let's look around".

When the child spots something or touches something, the therapist should prompt him/her to say, "Look therapist's name, it's a ...". Or "See my...." or "I have a ...". The therapist should try to vary these prompts and then fade them quickly.

The therapist should make comments about whatever the child shows the therapist, For example, "Oh, I see it has a purple dress. It has yellow hair". This should be repeated several times with different objects.

On a walk, at the park, in the grocery store, or at a restaurant:

The drill is the same as above. The therapist says, "Let's look for things." Then the therapist models the drill by saying, "John look! See the bird. It's blue." Then she says, "Your turn" and prompts. For example, "(therapist's name), look...." or "Look, (therapist's name)".

Information from school to talk about at home:

The child should choose one thing to bring home to show the parents each day. The child should choose what it will be -- it can be a work page, or craft, a book. Just about anything the child chooses will work.

When the child comes home, s/he should be prompted to say, "Look mom, I did this/I made this. It's a ...". The parent can then ask the child questions about whatever it is, but the key is to get the child to draw the parent's attention to something she did or has.

Periodically, the child should be prompted to show the therapist something s/he did at school as well. This will give the child additional practice. If the child goes to the store to buy something special, the therapist should make a point to have the child show someone what it is.

 # Why Teach Joint Attention?

The purpose of joint attention is to develop the child's ability to draw other people's attention to things that s/he finds are interesting or important. This is a good activity to do on a daily basis. The goal is to have the child internalize the process of getting other people to notice things the child cares about so the skill becomes part of the child's social repertoire.

How To Teach Contingent Statements

Spontaneous conversation is very difficult to teach because, by its very nature, it has no fixed format. It is loosely structured and spontaneous. This drill is an attempt to teach various structures of spontaneous speech. By doing these drills in order, from Step 1 to Step 5, the objective is for the child to become sufficiently comfortable with the various structures that they become internalized and are eventually used for truly spontaneous speech. An example of a contingent statement is: I LIKE TO EAT PIZZA. PIZZA HAS PEPPERONI.

Introductory Step: Comments and questions can be introduced using the "Making Comments & Asking Questions" sheet. This sheet is important because it gives the child a visual representation of comments and questions.

Step One: A good way to first introduce this drill is with a computer word processor, if possible. First, the therapist types a comment and the child is then given the opportunity to type a related comment. At first, this drill may have to be heavily prompted; however, the minute the child is able to understand the structure of the drill, it should go quite quickly, without prompts. Once the drill is understood using the computer, then the child and therapist should do the drill orally. The therapist makes a comment and the child must return a comment relating to the original comment. When the child becomes good at this, the next step is to make several contingent statements in a row (so the comments are made by: therapist, child, therapist, child, therapist, child). Once the child can answer the therapist's comment with a comment, then the child is taught to make the first comment (so the comments are made by: child, therapist, child, therapist, child, therapist). Only when the child masters Step One, should s/he go on to step two. Examples of the structure of the drill follow.

Step Two: In this variation, the therapist makes a comment, and the child makes a related comment. Then the child must ask a question related to the topic. At first, the therapist may have to prompt for the question (either orally or in written form). After the child learns this pattern, the prompts will be unnecessary. Once the child becomes good at this drill, step three should be introduced.

Step Three: The pattern for this drill is that the therapist makes a comment and then the child must ask the therapist a question. Then the therapist answers. The child must then ask another question related to the therapist's answer.

Problems: Step Three can be difficult for many children because the child is used to following immediately apparent structured patterns. With this step, the child must learn to listen to the comment, and then come up with a question rather than a comment. Prompting should help the child complete the exercise until s/he understands the structure of Step Three.

Step Four: In this variation, the therapist asks the child a question. The child answers the question and makes a comment related to his/her answer. Then the therapist asks the child a question related to the comment and the child answers.

Step Five: This is the most difficult variation of this drill, and the most similar to a natural spontaneous conversation. The child asks a question and the therapist responds. Then the child makes a comment related to the therapist's response and asks another question related to the topic.

Note: It is a bad idea to mix these drills until the child is very good at each of them since it is complicated enough to learn the pattern of each drill by itself. The goal is not for the child to become proficient in discerning one drill from the next; rather, these drills are meant to have the child become comfortable in speaking when presented with a variety of sequences and types of interchanges. Therefore, it is wise to do each drill in the order that it is presented and not to be in a hurry to complete the entire drill sequence. This sequence can take a long time to complete and once completed, the conversational practice should be used in speech. The conversation cards are a good way to maintain this skill.

Why Teach Contingent Statements?

Contingent statements are very important because they are the foundation of all conversation. Contingent statements, in their various forms, are necessary to teach because they help work on spontaneous speech, and are a precursor to elaborative statements which are a necessary part of conversation.

Making Comments and Asking Questions

Once the child is good at doing the contingent word exercise, it is time to introduce contingent statements. Making comments and asking questions are basic contingent statements introduced in this drill. The child must use the verb in the parenthesis to make a comment. Then the therapist must write the question she is going to ask the child and then ask the child (e.g. "John, what do you like to eat?"). Then the child must answer the therapist. Once the child understands the relationship between the verb and the question, the child can ask the therapist a question based on the therapist's question (e.g. "Therapist's name, what do you like to eat?"). This introductory drill is visual, so the child can grasp the structure of the comment and question.

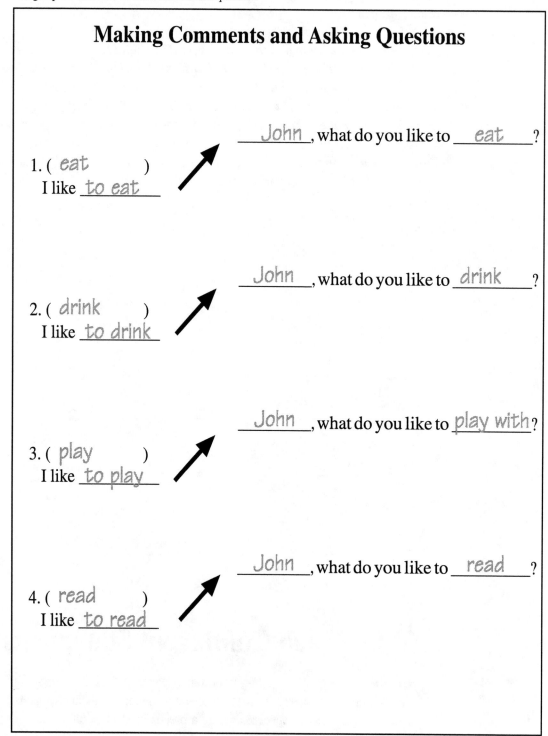

Making Comments and Asking Questions

1. (eat   )
   I like to eat

   ___John___ , what do you like to ___eat___ ?

2. (drink   )
   I like to drink

   ___John___ , what do you like to ___drink___ ?

3. (play   )
   I like to play

   ___John___ , what do you like to play with ?

4. (read   )
   I like to read

   ___John___ , what do you like to ___read___ ?

Samples of Contingent Statements

These are examples of the various steps of the contingent statement exercise that the child should go through. It is important to stay on each level until the child understands how to do the level well. This exercise is one that the child will be doing for years since it is so important in developing the child's ability to converse. The drill should be done daily at an appropriate level for the child. In order to bring the child to the level where Step 1, Comment - comment, can be taught, the child should be taught the contingent word exercise first.

STEP 1: Comment - Comment

Therapist: " I like to go to the beach."
Child: "I like to swim in the ocean."   ◄—————— COMMENT
Therapist: "The ocean has big waves."
Child: "I see dolphins in the ocean."   ◄—————— COMMENT
Therapist: "There are lots of fish in the ocean."

STEP 2: Comment - Question

Therapist: "It's fun to go on a picnic at the park."
Child: "I like to play in the sand at the park." ◄—————— COMMENT
Child: "What's your favorite thing to do at the park?" ◄—— QUESTION
Therapist: " I like to go down the slide."

STEP 3: Question - Question

Therapist: "I like to watch T.V."
Child: "What's your favorite video?"   ◄—————— QUESTION
Therapist: "My favorite video is 'The Lion King."
Child: "Did you like Aladdin?"   ◄—————— QUESTION
Therapist: "Yeah, Aladdin was good too."

STEP 4: Answer - Comment

Therapist: "Have you ever been to Disneyland?"
Child: "Yeah."   ◄—————————— ANSWER
Child: "I liked 'Pirates of the Caribbean!" ◄—— COMMENT
Therapist: "What about it's a Small World.
          Did you like that ride?"
Child: "Yeah, that was fun."

Samples of Contingent Statements (Continued)

STEP 5: Question - Comment - Question

Child: "What do you like to order at McDonald's?" ◄— QUESTION
Therapist: "I like to order a Happy Meal and a Coke."
Child: "I like Happy Meals too." ◄————— COMMENT
Child: "Do you like hamburgers or cheeseburgers?" ◄— QUESTION
Therapist: "I like the Filet of Fish in my Happy Meal."

 ## Conversation Cards

These are reproducible cards to be used as explained on the previous pages. They can be photocopied onto card stock to ensure their durability.

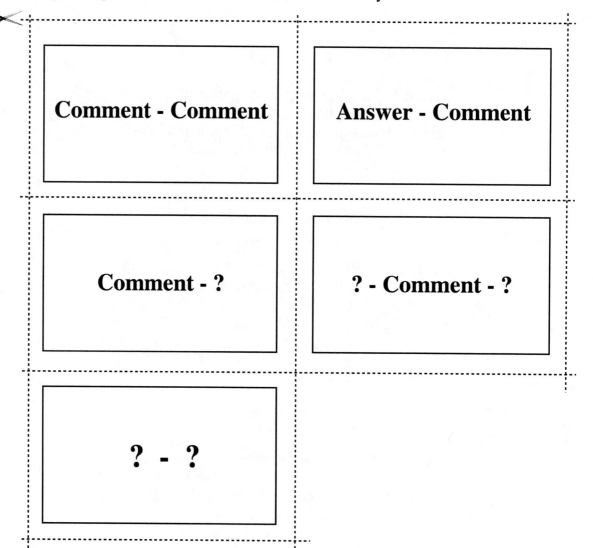

Comment - Comment

Answer - Comment

Comment - ?

? - Comment - ?

? - ?

How To Teach Conversation

The therapist begins this exercise by having the child come up with a variety of questions about the topic that has been chosen. At first the therapist should choose a topic that the child can ask many questions about; eventually, the child can choose the topic. Once the therapist has written down all the child's questions on the left side of the sheet, then the therapist should have the child answer the questions and the therapist should record them. Once the top part of the form is completed, then the entire conversation should be rehearsed using the sheet. Finally, the sheet should be removed and the child and therapist should have the actual conversation. This should be recorded by the therapist for comparison purposes.

It is important to make sure that the comments and questions relate to each other. To ensure that a variety of questions are asked, the therapist can prompt the child to ask a What, Where, Who, or Which question. Eventually, the child should be able to vary the questions on his/her own.

The "Conversational Self-Monitoring" form is a way for the child to keep track of his/her part of the conversation. It also shifts the responsibility to keep the conversation going from the conversant (the therapist, adult or peer) to the child.

Why Teach Conversation This Way?

This is another way to teach the child the structure of a conversation. Some children will recognize that a conversation is composed of related questions and comments, whereas other children will understand the components of a conversation better if they see one in its entire state.

Topical Questions/Comments For Conversation

This exercise structures a conversation using Who, What, Where, and Which questions. The child's responses must be written down because it should help him/her stay on task and see how the questions and responses relate to the topic. Questions that simply require a Yes or No answer should be avoided unless the child is going to expand a Yes or No answer. The therapist should NOT require the child to answer a yes or no question in a full sentence **every time** because the child will sound stilted. Children rarely answer yes or no questions in a full sentence. The actual conversation that takes place should be written down as it is happening, so 1) the child can see the conversation after it has taken place, and 2) the therapist has a record of comparison for future progress checks.

Topical Questions/Comments For Conversation

Topic: ___The Beach___

Questions I can ask:

Do you like the beach?

What do you like to do at the beach?

Who do you like to go to the beach with?

Which beach do you like to go to?

Comments I can make:

I like the beach.

I like to build sand castles

I like to go with my friends.

I like to go to Santa Cruz beach

Actual Conversation: (Rehearse above in Question - Response format with the therapist asking the question., Then talk about the beach without a visual prompt, and record below).

Do you like the beach?   Yeah, I do like the beach. What do you like to do at the beach? ... build sand castles.   Who goes to the beach with you? ... my friends.   Which beach do you like to go to the most? I like to go to the Santa Cruz beach.

Conversational Self-Monitoring

This form is designed to have the child monitor his/her own conversation. First, the child chooses a topic. S/he begins with either a question or a comment, and then asks a question. The therapist then answers the question. The child must either make a comment or ask a question to keep the conversation going. Every time the child makes a new statement (question or comment - question) s/he puts an X in the box. The child must keep the conversation going for at least 8 exchanges. The child uses the top row if s/he asks a question, and the second row if s/he makes a comment.

Conversation Self-Monitoring

My job: Keep the conversation going through at least 8 turns by asking questions and making comments.

TOPIC: Instruments   [X] [X] [ ] [X] **?**

[X] [X] [X] [ ] **C**

Summary of Conversation: What's your favorite instrument? Piano. I like the piano. Do you like the electric guitar? Yeah. I like the beatles. My favorite song is Yellow Submarine. I like the drums. I like the drums. Do you like the trumpet? Yeah, it's ok.

TOPIC: movies   [X] [X] [X] [X] **?**

[X] [ ] [ ] [ ] **C**

Summary of Conversation: What's your favorite movie? Babe. I liked Pocahontas. Do you like Pocahontas. No, It was too scary.. Do you like Lion King. Yeah, I did. I liked the Lion. Do you like the Little Mermaid? Yeah, I liked Ariel.

? = question

C = comment

Having A Conversation

The conversation script is designed to give the child an idea of the purpose, the various parts and the structure of a conversation. This script attempts to make explicit the implicit nature of a conversation and should be read with the child often over a period of time so the child becomes very familiar with the script. The therapist should discuss the script with the child asking questions such as, "What can you talk about in a conversation?"

Having A Conversation

Having a CONVERSATION with people is VERY IMPORTANT.
Having a CONVERSATION means TALKING WITH SOMEONE.
When you have a CONVERSATION with someone, you TALK ABOUT A TOPIC.

TALKING ABOUT A TOPIC means TALKING ABOUT AN IDEA.
Here are some TOPICS and IDEAS you can have a CONVERSATION about.
You can TALK ABOUT:
- Your favorite movie
- What you like to eat
- Where you like to go
- Your family
- A TV show you watched
- Something you did that was fun
- Sports, like basketball or baseball

When you have a CONVERSATION with someone, you TAKE TURNS TALKING ABOUT THE TOPIC.

Here is a CONVERSATION between Sue and Stacey ABOUT MOVIES.
Sue: *"I love going to movies, do you?"*
Stacey: *"Yeah, I like it a lot. I just saw Pocahontas. Did you see that movie?"*
Sue: *"No, I haven't seen it yet, but I really want to see Pocahontas!"*

When you have a CONVERSATION about a topic, you can MAKE A COMMENT.
When you make a COMMENT, you SAY SOMETHING ABOUT THE TOPIC.
"I just saw Pocahontas" is a COMMENT.
"But I really want to see Pocahontas "is a COMMENT.

When you have a CONVERSATION about a topic, you can also ASK A QUESTION.
"Do you like going to movies?" is a QUESTION.
"Did you see that movie?" is a QUESTION.

When you have a CONVERSATION, you need to DO THESE THINGS:

- LOOK AT THE PERSON you are talking to.
- LISTEN to what your talking partner is saying.
- TALK ABOUT THE TOPIC your partner is talking about.
- MAKE COMMENTS and ASK QUESTIONS about the topic.
- KEEP THE CONVERSATION GOING.

Having a CONVERSATION with people is VERY IMPORTANT.
You should TRY TO HAVE LOTS OF CONVERSATIONS with people EVERY DAY.

Conversation Equations

Conversation equations should be introduced to the child immediately after the child goes through the "Having a Conversation" script. The child should read the equations aloud and then be asked questions about having a conversation. For example, the child should be asked "Having a conversation means _____"; "Talking ON Topic means _____"; "Talking OFF topic means _____".

Conversation Equations

HAVING A = TALKING = TALKING ABOUT A TOPIC = MAKING COMMENTS
CONVERSATION   WITH   AND ASKING QUESTIONS
                            SOMEONE   ABOUT THE TOPIC

TALKING ON = TALKING ABOUT THE TOPIC = MAKING AN ON TOPIC = GOOD
TOPIC   COMMENT   CONVERSATION

TALKING OFF = NOT TALKING ABOUT = MAKING AN OFF TOPIC = NOT A GOOD
THE TOPIC   TOPIC   COMMENT   CONVERSATION

Conversation Games

Tell Me Five Things About...

In this conversation game, each player must say five things about the topic he chooses from a pile of topic cards (provided in Chapter 4 accompanying the WH Game). The therapist goes first and models the game. Let's say she chooses elephants from the pile. The therapist must name five things about an elephant. It is a good idea if she uses her fingers to count off each thing while listing them. When the child has his/her turn, the therapist should prompt the child by having the child use his/her fingers to do the same thing. Often, the use of the child's fingers to prompt 5 things helps the child give full sentences to describe the topic.

The first few times this game is played, it is a good idea for the therapist to give the child only topics that s/he knows a lot about. In this way, the game will flow and the structure of the game will become clear before the game becomes more challenging. The therapist and the child should take turns, with the therapist using topics that are slightly challenging for the child. In this way, the child learns to pay attention to oral information that has not been completely internalized.

Ask Me About ...

To play this game, the therapist needs a spinner (like the one below) and a list of topics that are of interest to the child. Examples of topics of interest include fast-food restaurants, toys or characters such as Disney or Ninja Turtle characters, games, and videos. First the therapist chooses the topic and then the child spins the spinner. Whatever question the spinner lands on, the child must ask that question about the topic. So, for example, if the topic is Mickey Mouse, and the spinner lands on "Why", the child must ask a "Why" question such as, "Why do you like Mickey Mouse?", or "Why does Mickey Mouse have big ears?" Other questions the child could ask, depending upon where the spinner lands are:
"What does Mickey have on his head?"
"Where does Mickey live?"
"When did you see Mickey?"
"Who did you see Mickey with?"
"How do you go to the disney store (or Disneyland)?"

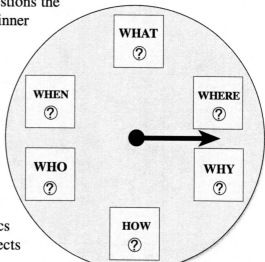

The more topics of interest the therapist can think of, the better the drill will be for the child. Exposure to a large number of topics will increase the number and variety of subjects the child can discuss.

How To Teach Emotions

The following emotion scripts are only examples of scripts that can be written. It is important to take each script and customize it to the child since what makes one child happy may make another child sad. It is crucial the script be relevant to the child in order for the child to be helped by this drill. Otherwise, the child might become confused.

It is important to start with the four basic emotions of happy, sad, mad and scared. Even if the child may understand these emotions, these scripts should be completed with the child. It is easier for the child to become familiarized with the script format when teaching easy emotions than when teaching difficult, abstract emotions.

1. The script must be written in the form of the first person ("I" form). This relates the script directly to the child and makes it easier to comprehend. The emotions must be taught from the child's perspective. This is IMPORTANT!
2. Once the child has comprehended the emotion from the child's point of view (the "I" perspective), then this same emotion should be introduced from other significant people's perspectives (e.g. what makes Mom or Dad feel happy). This technique is designed to train the child to see things from another person's point of view, and is critical to the child's ability to understand that others can feel, think, and behave differently.

There are a large number of emotions that are not clear cut, such as proud, frustrated, and worried. The therapist may be identifying a feeling that has never been labelled for the child. Since this emotion may be new, it is best written from the "you" global perspective (e.g. You can feel proud of your family). The scripts provide examples of situations or events that might bring on these emotions. The more abstract emotions are difficult to delineate for any given child; therefore, they must be customized to the child and introduced gradually.

It is important to remember that each child is unique in his/her ability to understand emotions. Some children may be unable to fully grasp the concepts of pride or anxiety, for example. At minimum, however, all children should be introduced to the emotions of happiness, sadness, anger, and fear.

If possible, the therapist should pair the script with actual pictures of the child "caught" in situations that illustrate the emotion being taught. Overlapping the visual picture with the written words will significantly increase most children's comprehension of the emotion.

In addition, when the child is expressing an emotion (e.g. crying), the person with the child should label that emotion and give a reason why the child is emotional (e.g. "You're feeling sad because ...").

Why Teach Emotions?

Emotions are very difficult to teach because so many of them are subtle. Therefore, it is important to make them as explicit as possible in order for the child to understand how they relate to him/her. Most children pick up subtle emotions from the natural environment; however, these children often do not pick up the labels which correspond to the feelings they have. For example, children with developmental delays most probably feel frustration equally as often (if not more often) than their normally developing peers; however, their way of coping with the emotion may be socially unacceptable, whereas, their normally developing peers can express that emotion in a more appropriate manner. These drills attempt to give children with language delays the skills to identify and label their feelings and express these feelings in a manner that is socially acceptable.

Feeling Happy

The Feeling Happy script is the first emotion script that should be introduced. The child and the therapist should alternate reading lines in the script. This script should be read with the child every day for a week or two (until the child knows the script well). During this time, the child should be asked questions about the emotion. For example, the therapist should ask, "What makes you happy?", and the child should name a few things that makes him/her happy. The child can use items written in the script (since the script is customized to reflect the child's feelings the items should be accurate); however, s/he can also suggest new things. The script should be used when "Happy" is first introduced. Eventually, the script should be removed and the emotion "Happy" should be discussed orally. The equation at the bottom should be reviewed several times as well.

Feeling Happy

When I am HAPPY, I FEEL GOOD.
When I am HAPPY, I FEEL GLAD.

There are MANY THINGS THAT CAN MAKE ME HAPPY.
 EATING ICE CREAM makes me HAPPY.
 PLAYING WITH TRAINS makes me HAPPY.
 WATCHING VIDEOS makes me HAPPY.
 SWINGING AT THE PARK makes me HAPPY.
 GETTING HUGS AND KISSES FROM MOM makes me HAPPY.

When I am HAPPY, I SMILE AND LAUGH.

There are MANY THINGS that I CAN DO TO MAKE OTHER PEOPLE HAPPY
 When I PLAY AND SHARE WITH MY FRIENDS, I MAKE MOM HAPPY
 When I PLAY THE PIANO NICELY, I MAKE MOM HAPPY.
 When I DO ALL MY WORK AT SCHOOL, I MAKE MY TEACHER HAPPY.
 When I TALK TO DAD, I MAKE DAD HAPPY.

When I make other people HAPPY, THEY FEEL GOOD.
When I make other people HAPPY, THEY FEEL GLAD.

IT IS IMPORTANT TO FEEL HAPPY.
IT IS IMPORTANT TO MAKE OTHER PEOPLE FEEL HAPPY.

Feeling Happy Equation

FEELING HAPPY = FEELING GOOD = FEELING GLAD

Feeling Sad

The Feeling Sad script is the second emotion script that should be introduced. The child and the therapist should alternate reading lines in the script. This script should be read with the child every day for a week or two (until the child knows the script well). During this time, the child should be asked questions about the emotion similar in structure to the questions asked for the Happy script. The equation at the bottom should be reviewed several times as well.

Feeling Sad

When I am SAD, I FEEL BAD.
When I am SAD, I DON'T FEEL HAPPY.

There are MANY THINGS THAT CAN MAKE ME SAD.
     I get SAD when I LOSE MY FAVORITE DOLL.
     I get SAD when I GET HURT.
     I get SAD when I MOM OR DAD YELLS AT ME.
     I get SAD when I CAN'T FIND MY MOM.

When I am SAD, sometimes I CRY.
When I am SAD and I CRY, a HUG from mom or dad MAKES ME
FEEL BETTER.

When I AM SAD, it is IMPORTANT that I let mom or dad know why I am SAD.
I need to TELL THEM OR SHOW THEM WHY I AM SAD.

WHEN I TELL MOM AND DAD WHY I AM SAD, THEY CAN HELP
ME FEEL BETTER.

Feeling Sad Equation

FEELING SAD = FEELING BAD = NOT FEELING HAPPY

Feeling Mad

The Feeling Mad script should be introduced after Happy and Sad. The child and the therapist should alternate reading lines in the script. This script should be read with the child every day for a week or two (until the child knows the script well). During this time, the child should be asked questions about the emotion similar in structure to the questions asked for the two preceding scripts. The equation at the bottom should be reviewed several times as well.

Feeling Mad

When I am MAD, I FEEL ANGRY.

There are MANY THINGS THAT CAN MAKE ME MAD.
     I get MAD when I CAN'T PLAY WITH MY LETTERS.
     I get MAD when I CAN'T HAVE CANDY.
     I get MAD when MOM BRUSHES MY TEETH.
     I get MAD when JANE TAKES MY TRAINS.

When I am MAD, sometimes I CRY.
When I am MAD, sometimes I SCREAM.
When I am MAD, sometimes I HIT AND THROW THINGS.

When I AM MAD, it is IMPORTANT that I let mom or dad know why I am MAD.
I need to TELL THEM OR SHOW THEM WHY I AM MAD.

WHEN I AM MAD, I SHOULD NOT SCREAM OR HIT OR THROW THINGS.
WHEN I AM MAD, I NEED TO TALK ABOUT WHY I AM MAD.
IT'S O.K. TO BE MAD, BUT IT'S NOT O.K. TO SCREAM OR HIT OR THROW THINGS.

Feeling Mad Equation

FEELING MAD = FEELING ANGRY

Feeling Scared

The Feeling Scared script should be introduced once the child really understands the idea of emotions. If the child has not internalized the first three, it may be a good idea to wait a while before scared is introduced. Scared is a much more difficult emotion for some children to grasp than happy, or sad. The child and the therapist should alternate reading lines in the script. This script should be read with the child every day for a week or two (until the child knows the script well). During this time, the child should be asked questions about the emotion similar in structure to the questions asked for the preceding scripts. The equation at the bottom should be gone over several times as well.

Feeling Scared

When I am SCARED, I FEEL AFRAID.

There are MANY THINGS THAT CAN MAKE ME SCARED.
>   I get SCARED when IT IS DARK.
>   I get SCARED when I HEAR THE VACUUM CLEANER.
>   I get SCARED when I AM SWINGING AND MY FEET ARE OFF
>   THE GROUND.
>   I get SCARED when I HEAR A SIREN.

When I am SCARED, sometimes I CRY.
When I am SCARED, sometimes I SCREAM.
When I am SCARED, sometimes I RUN AND HIDE.

When I AM SCARED, I WANT MY MOM.
When I AM SCARED, I WANT MY MOM TO HOLD ME TIGHT.

When I am SCARED, it is IMPORTANT to let mom or dad know why I am SCARED.
I need to TELL MOM OR SHOW MOM WHY I AM SCARED.

Feeling Scared Equation

FEELING SCARED = FEELING AFRAID = FEELING FRIGHTENED

Feeling Proud

The Feeling Proud script should be introduced once the child really understands the idea of emotions. Some children never internalize the feeling of proud which is okay. There are other more important areas to concentrate on besides abstract emotions. If the child is not ready, it is a good idea to wait for the child to mature and try to introduce the emotion in a year. If the child has difficulty even after s/he matures, it is a good idea to move on. If the child is ready, then the script should be introduced in the same way as the other scripts. The equation at the bottom should be gone over several times as well. The reader should notice that this script is written in the "you" global perspective.

Feeling Proud

When you are PROUD, you FEEL GOOD ABOUT SOMETHING YOU HAVE.
When you are PROUD, you FEEL GOOD ABOUT SOMETHING YOU HAVE DONE.

When you feel PROUD , you FEEL HAPPY.
When you feel PROUD , you FEEL GOOD ABOUT YOURSELF.

These are SOME THINGS YOU CAN FEEL PROUD ABOUT.
    You can feel PROUD ABOUT A NEW BIKE.
    You can feel PROUD OF YOUR FAMILY.
    You can feel PROUD ABOUT READING AND FINISHING A LONG BOOK.
    You can feel PROUD ABOUT WRITING A STORY.
    You can feel PROUD ABOUT DOING GOOD WORK.
    You can feel PROUD ABOUT FINISHING YOUR HOMEWORK.
    You can feel PROUD ABOUT ANSWERING A HARD QUESTION.

Other people can be PROUD OF YOU.
When other people are PROUD OF YOU, they are HAPPY THAT YOU DID SOMETHING.

These are SOME THINGS THAT MAKE OTHER PEOPLE PROUD OF YOU.
Other people are PROUD OF YOU WHEN:

    You LISTEN AND PAY ATTENTION.
    You DO YOUR WORK.
    You TRY TO DO SOMETHING THAT IS HARD FOR YOU TO DO.
    You RAISE YOUR HAND AND ANSWER QUESTIONS.
    You TALK AND PLAY WITH KIDS.
    You FOLLOW THE RULES.
    You ACT LIKE A BIG KID.

Feeling PROUD is a NICE FEELING.
Feeling PROUD makes you FEEL GOOD ABOUT YOURSELF.

Having OTHER PEOPLE FEEL PROUD OF YOU, is a NICE FEELING, TOO.
Having OTHER PEOPLE FEEL PROUD OF YOU, makes you FEEL HAPPY.

Your mom, dad, grandma, grandpa, teachers, Debbie, and Jan ARE ALL PROUD OF YOU.
Doing things that MAKE OTHER PEOPLE PROUD OF YOU is GOOD.
Doing things that MAKE OTHER PEOPLE PROUD OF YOU is IMPORTANT.

Feeling Proud Equation

FEELING PROUD = FEELING GOOD = MAKES YOU HAPPY = MAKES YOU FEEL GOOD = IS IMPORTANT
    ABOUT SOMETHING   ABOUT YOURSELF
    YOU HAVE OR SOME-
    THING YOU
    HAVE DONE

Feeling Frustrated

The Frustrated script should be introduced once the child really understands the idea of emotions. Some children cannot differentiate between mad and frustrated which is not a critical differentiation to make. If the child is ready, then the script should be introduced in the same way as the other scripts. The equation at the bottom should be reviewed several times as well.

Feeling Frustrated

When I CAN'T DO SOMETHING I WANT TO DO, I FEEL FRUSTRATED.

There are MANY THINGS THAT CAN MAKE ME FRUSTRATED.
I get FRUSTRATED when I CAN'T TIE MY SHOES.
I get FRUSTRATED when I CAN'T ZIP UP MY JACKET.
I get FRUSTRATED when I CAN'T RIDE MY TWO-WHEEL BIKE.
I get FRUSTRATED when I CAN'T FIND MY FAVORITE GAME ON THE
    COMPUTER.
I get FRUSTRATED when I TRY TO DO MY MATH BUT IT'S TOO HARD.

When I am FRUSTRATED, I GET UPSET.
When I am FRUSTRATED, sometimes I CRY.
When I am FRUSTRATED, sometimes I GET MAD.
When I am FRUSTRATED, sometimes I SCREAM.

When I AM FRUSTRATED, it is IMPORTANT TO LET MOM OR DAD
KNOW WHY I AM FRUSTRATED.
I need to TELL MOM OR SHOW MOM WHAT I NEED HELP WITH.

WHEN I SHOW MOM WHAT I AM FRUSTRATED WITH, SHE CAN
HELP ME DO THE THING I WANT TO DO.

Feeling Frustrated Equation

FEELING FRUSTRATED = CAN'T DO SOMETHING = MAKES YOU UPSET
YOU WANT TO DO

How To Use The Emotions Sheet

After the child is familiar with their own happy, sad, and mad emotions, the parents and therapist must each complete a Mad, Happy, Sad sheet which the therapist then uses to create the drills for emotions (see the completed Emotions Sheet). The first step is to have the person closest to the child - usually the mother - make a list of situations/things that make her happy, sad, and mad. The situations should include the child as a component (e.g. I am happy when John pays attention. I am sad when John gets hurt, etc.). The list becomes the therapist's working list in which she can write the various situations in the exercises. The following activity sheets "Determining A Cause", "Identifying Situations - Emotions-Consequences" and "Identifying People's Reactions and Providing Solutions", must be customized to the child based on the Mad, Happy, Sad sheet. The therapist should begin by reading the list with the child, starting with one feeling at a time e.g. "I am (or "Mom is") happy when John does his work"; I am happy when John plays with his friends". To focus the child, the adult should point to the word "mom", point to "feeling happy", and then read the situation the emotion refers to. The adult should continue through the list, focusing on only one feeling at a time. Next, the child should verbalize the list e.g. "Mom is happy when I do work", replacing the child's name with I (the therapist can do this with the child as well). Once the list is reviewed, the adult should start using the cause-effect drills e.g. "John did his work. How did mom feel?" or "Mom is happy when John _____". It is important to use the list of situations in as many cause-effect drills as possible.

1. Determining A Cause (see the completed exercise)
This activity sheet should be filled in by the therapist based on the Mad, Happy, Sad sheets completed by the therapist and/or parents. Then the therapist should read this exercise with the child and have the child answer the questions. At first, the child may not be clear about how to answer so the therapist should prompt the child. Once the child understands the structure of the drill, then the therapist can fade out the prompts.

2. Identifying Situations - Emotions - Consequences (see the completed exercise)
This activity should also be based on the Mad, Happy, Sad sheet and introduced to the child after the Determining A Cause drill has been done many times. The therapist should read the sheet with the child and try to show (using arrows) the obvious causes of the emotions.

3. Problems: Identifying People's Reactions and Providing Solutions (see the completed exercise)
Prerequisite: Before introducing this third "Emotions" exercise, the child should be introduced to the "Problem/Solution" exercises which follow.
This is the most complex of the activities working on emotions. The therapist should read through this sheet with the child and have the child answer all the questions asked, thereby identifying the problem and its solution. This may be difficult at first; however, after a while, the child should be able to do this drill using the sheet. Once s/he can answer all the questions while looking at the sheet, the therapist should ask the child to identify people's reactions and provide "solutions" to problems in real life situations without the sheet.

Why Teach Emotions This Way?

Children with developmental disorders often find themselves breaking social rules, quite unaware that they are doing anything wrong. These drills attempt to structure the behavior problems that cause the child trouble. The sheets attempt to teach the child to identify the problem behavior and come up with a solution, thereby giving the child the opportunity to gain some control in the interaction. It is also a highly structured way of discussing every problem that may arise, having the child identify potential problems, and then offering a solution. The drills teach the child how feelings are experienced by someone else - those people he is most familiar with. In effect, we are trying to teach the child how to see/ experience emotions from another's viewpoint.

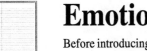

Emotions Sheet

Before introducing any of the "Emotion, Cause and Effect" exercises, the mother, father or therapist should complete this sheet. Then the child should listen to the person read one of the emotion columns. It is a good idea to work on happy first. After a few sessions, the next emotion should be chosen. The child is simply being introduced to the emotions and will probably not gain a full understanding from this sheet; however, the sheet should be used to create the following exercises. Through those exercises the child will begin to gain an idea of how we label feelings.

Emotions Sheet

(Mom, Dad or name of therapist)

Things that make me MAD	**Things that make me HAPPY**	**Things that make me SAD**
I get mad when...	*I am happy when...*	*I am sad when...*
John does not listen to the teacher	John plays piano well	John cries
John sings during lessons	John talks to me	John is sad
John acts weird	John plays nicely with his friends	John is sick
John pinches	John listens to to the teacher	John does not want listen to me
John drinks from the faucet	John acts nice at gymnastics	I have to yell at John

Determining A Cause

This is the first exercise that makes explicit the relationship between events that the child causes and the emotional reactions to those events. It is very difficult to take these explicit relationships and have the child internalize them; however, it is important that the child have some sense that s/he can cause or avoid situations which create undesired emotions e.g. anger or sadness. This sheet must be customized to the child to make it relevant.

Determining A Cause

Event/Situation	Cause/Why? How?
Suzie did not listen to Mom.	How did Mom feel?
	Why was Mom mad?

When the child becomes good at this drill, add: What would make Mom Happy? or What can you do to make Mom happy?

Suzie paid attention in school.	How did Mom feel?
	Why was Mom happy?
Suzie was sick.	How did Mom feel?
	Why was Mom sad?

With a negative situation, the therapist can ask a question such as: "What can/should you do to make Mom feel better?"

Identifying Situations: Emotions/ Consequences

This exercise defines the role of emotions in social interaction. It makes explicit what is generally implicit and obvious to most normally developing children. The sheets need to be customized to the child's actions and behaviors, and the resultant emotions from those behaviors.

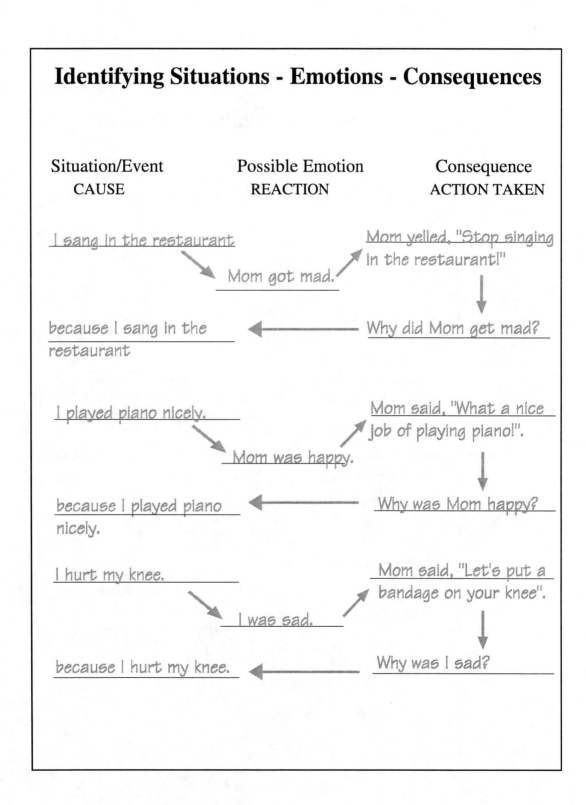

Identifying Situations - Emotions - Consequences

Situation/Event CAUSE	Possible Emotion REACTION	Consequence ACTION TAKEN
I sang in the restaurant	Mom got mad.	Mom yelled, "Stop singing in the restaurant!"
because I sang in the restaurant		Why did Mom get mad?
I played piano nicely.	Mom was happy.	Mom said, "What a nice job of playing piano!".
because I played piano nicely.		Why was Mom happy?
I hurt my knee.	I was sad.	Mom said, "Let's put a bandage on your knee".
because I hurt my knee.		Why was I sad?

Problems, People's Reactions & Solutions

This exercise teaches the relationship between events and people's emotional reactions. The child needs to know why people become angry with him/her and how the child can prevent or decrease the number of unpleasant episodes. This sheet must be customized to the child using situations in which the child 1) makes someone angry; and 2) makes someone sad.

Problems: Identifying People's Reactions and Providing Solutions

Read about each situation, then answer the questions.

You're in class and Mrs. Howard asks you a question.

You are not paying attention to the question.

| What is/was the problem? | I am not paying attention. |

| Who or what caused the problem? | Me | Who did the problem affect or bother? | Mrs. Howard |

| How did it affect Mrs. Howard ? | She feels angry. |

| How can the problem be solved? | SOLUTION: I should stop and I should pay attention to Mrs. Howard. |

| How else can the problem be solved? | ANOTHER SOLUTION: |

How To Teach Critical Thinking

The following is the most effective sequence for the therapist to use when reviewing a script with a child:

1. First the lines of the script should be read with the child, emphasizing key words. Having the child read every second line keeps him/her focused.

2. Second, the therapist should read the key statements from the script, leaving out key words for the child to fill-in verbally. For example, the therapist can say, "Something dangerous is something that can _____" or, "Something dangerous causes _____." The verbal fill-in technique encourages the child to pay close attention while working on the script. Once the child understands the exercise, the script should be removed and the child should answer the questions verbally (without a visual prompt).

3. Next, the therapist should ask questions about the script having the script in full view so the child can refer back it to if s/he cannot answer the question. An example of a question to ask from a script would be, "Is playing the piano safe or dangerous?"

4. Finally, the therapist should remove the script and have the child answer the command: "Tell me what you know about _____."

The scripts should be introduced one at a time and should be accompanied by the corresponding equation and activity sheets. Once the child has become very good at the script and activity sheets that follow the script (generally after weeks of working on one script) then the therapist can introduce another script. Once all the scripts have been exhausted, the therapist should create new scripts that address a critical thinking issue in the child's life. Since every child is different, each script should be customized.

The first topic is "Safe and Dangerous". The script should be introduced as explained in the above 1 through 4 steps. Then the Safe-Dangerous Equation should be read with the child. After several sessions of reading the script and equation, the "Identifying If A Situation Is Safe or Dangerous" sheet should be completed with the child. The child should be asked WHY the situation is Safe or Dangerous. This sheet should be given to the child with new situations each time until s/he understands these concepts. An understanding of Safe and Dangerous will take a very long time for many children due to the Why-Because relationship of Safe/Dangerous being applied to a variety of situations.

Once the child understands "Safe/Dangerous", then "Problems/Solutions" can be introduced. The script and equation should be introduced as described above. After the child acquires a sense of the meaning of Problem/Solution (which may take some time), the "Identifying If There is a Problem" sheet can be introduced. The situations given must be relevant to the child so that the problems chosen have some personal meaning i.e. if the child draws on the walls, this should be one of the problems s/he learns about.

The third topic is "Deciding Whom To Listen To". Children with autism spectrum disorders often follow directions from anyone, once they are taught to listen to instruction. For their personal safety and appropriate social behavior, these children must often be taught from whom they should follow directions. This script should be introduced as explained above. Then the therapist should work with the child on the "Deciding What To Do" sheet. The problem at the top of the sheet must always encompass a situation where someone tells the child to do something. The child then must evaluate the instruction. The therapist should help the child complete the sheet until s/he understands the structure of this exercise. Eventually, the child should be able to complete the sheet independently.

Note: It is important to include both positive and negative situations in the exercises, and instructions the child should and should not follow.

Why Teach Critical Thinking?

It is VERY IMPORTANT to teach critical thinking skills because children with developmental disorders do not necessarily pick up the subtleties present in many situations where critical thinking is crucial. Although these children may be naturally good problem solvers when they apply themselves, there are safety issues which need must be emphasized and critical thinking skills which must be developed. This section attempts to focus attention on general critical thinking skills that are sure to arise throughout the child's life. If the child can learn about these situations, it may make his/her life easier socially as well as enabling the child to start to take responsibility for his/her physical safety. It is crucial to work on dangerous situations well supervised, using the scripts as an tool to communicate to the child what is being required of him/her. It is a good idea to take ideas from the scripts and apply them to real life situation. For example, when in a parking lot the adult should ask the child, "Should we run to the store?". The child should then respond, "No, because running in the parking lot is dangerous."

NOTE: Some children are good at reciting the script back to the parent or therapist, but may not understand the TRUE danger being discussed. It is important to use the script as a starting point to teach critical thinking; however, the script alone will generally NOT teach the child to avoid danger. For example, crossing the street must be taught by behavioral professionals working with the child one-on-one actually on the street. Truly dangerous situations (such as crossing the street) may take years to teach!

Safe and Dangerous

The Safe and Dangerous script should be introduced to work on the child's critical thinking skills. The child and the therapist should alternate reading lines in the script. This script should be read with the child every day for a week or two (until the child knows the script well). During this time, the child should be asked questions so s/he can decide whether an action or situation is safe or dangerous.

Safe and Dangerous

Some things are SAFE and some things are DANGEROUS.

Something SAFE is something that WILL NOT HURT YOU.
YOU CAN DO THINGS THAT ARE SAFE.
There are lots of things that are SAFE.
These are some SAFE THINGS:

1. Playing the piano
2. Talking with friends
3. Tying your shoe
4. Listening to music
5. Eating food you like
6. Playing with dolls
7. Sleeping
8. Reading a book
9. Watching a video
10. Singing a song

Something DANGEROUS is something that CAN HURT YOU OR HARM YOU.
Something DANGEROUS causes TROUBLE.
Something DANGEROUS causes a PROBLEM.
YOU SHOULD NOT DO THINGS THAT ARE DANGEROUS.
There are lots of things that are DANGEROUS.
These are some DANGEROUS THINGS:

1. Running in the street
2. Running in the parking lot
3. Walking away from Mom or Dad at the store
4. Jumping off high things
5. Playing with matches
6. Not wearing your seat belt in the car
7. Not wearing your bike helmet while riding a bike
8. Getting too close to a fire
9. Eating things that are not food
10. Chewing on wires or cords

BEFORE I DO SOMETHING, I NEED TO DO THESE THINGS:

FIRST I NEED TO STOP AND THINK ABOUT WHAT I MIGHT DO,
THEN I NEED TO ASK MYSELF IF IT IS SAFE OR DANGEROUS,
LAST I NEED TO DECIDE WHAT TO DO.

I WILL NOT GET HURT IF I THINK AND DECIDE BEFORE I DO SOMETHING.

Safe Dangerous Equation

The child needs to know this equation very well. The therapist should have him/her review it verbally many times. The child should be prompted to say, "If something is safe, it will not hurt you; there is no problem, and you can do it." "If something is dangerous, it can hurt you; it is a problem, and you don't do it". The child should also be given some of the safe/dangerous situations that are listed on the safe/dangerous script to "plug" into this format. e.g. "Watching TV is safe. If will not hurt you. Watching TV is not a problem and you can do it." This will probably require prompting for a while, but it may be the quickest way to get the child to understand safe/dangerous by comparing these situations to each other. Note: the child will not truly understand Safe and Dangerous until s/he understands the concept of cause and effect.

Safe- Dangerous Comparison

SAFE = WILL NOT Hurt You = NO problem = You CAN do it

DANGEROUS = CAN Hurt You = Problem = You DO NOT do it

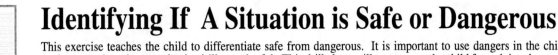

Identifying If A Situation is Safe or Dangerous

This exercise teaches the child to differentiate safe from dangerous. It is important to use dangers in the child's environment in order to make the drill meaningful. This drill alone will not prevent the child from doing dangerous activities; however, it will start to get the child to think about the categories of safe and dangerous. This drill is a good companion to actual safety training but will not replace intensive lessons on traffic safety, etc. Once the child identifies safe from dangerous, attempt to ask why something is safe or is dangerous. This part of the exercise will require much prompting because the child must have an understanding of Why/Because in order to answer the safety questions.

Identifying If A Situation is Safe or Dangerous

Read each sentence. If the sentence is talking about something dangerous, write "dangerous" on the line. If the sentence is talking about something safe, write "safe" on the line. The therapist should do this verbally once the child understands the format.

Situation

Playing the piano

Running in the street.
Why is running in the street dangerous?

Playing with matches
e.g. variation: playing with the lit candles on a birthday cake.

Watching a video

Jumping off high things
e.g. variation: jumping off the roof/jumping off the top of a slide

Safe Or Dangerous?

Safe
Because it will not hurt you. It's o.k.

Dangerous
Because, you could get hit by a car.

Dangerous
Because you could start a fire.

Safe
Because it will not hurt you.

Dangerous
Because you could hurt yourself.

Problems and Solutions

The Problem/Solution script is introduced to work on the child's critical thinking skills. The child and the therapist should alternate reading lines in the script. This script should be read with the child every day for many therapy sessions (until the child knows the script well). During this time, the child should be asked questions which may be the child decide whether an action or situation is a problem. Asking questions promotes understanding. The child must learn safe and dangerous well before introducing problem/solution. The therapist should make sure that the child understands that danger is always a problem, but a problem is not always dangerous.

Problems and Solutions

A PROBLEM is something that causes trouble.

You can have a PROBLEM BETWEEN YOURSELF AND ANOTHER PERSON.
You can have a PROBLEM WITH SOMETHING YOU ARE TRYING TO DO.
Sometimes, you can have a PROBLEM if you DON'T DO SOMETHING YOU SHOULD.

Here are some PROBLEMS you can have:

FIGHTING WITH A FRIEND is a PROBLEM. Fighting CAUSES TROUBLE.
NOT SHARING A TOY WITH YOUR FRIEND is a PROBLEM. Not sharing CAUSES TROUBLE.
DOING SOMETHING DANGEROUS is a PROBLEM. Dangerous things CAUSE TROUBLE.
MAKING FUN OF SOMEONE is a PROBLEM. Making fun of someone CAUSES TROUBLE.
NOT TALKING TO MOM AND DAD is a PROBLEM. Not talking CAUSES TROUBLE.
NOT DOING YOUR WORK is a PROBLEM. Not doing your work GETS YOU IN TROUBLE.
NOT LISTENING is a PROBLEM. Not listening GETS YOU IN TROUBLE.
SINGING TOO LOUDLY IN A RESTAURANT is a PROBLEM. It GETS YOU IN TROUBLE.

When you have a PROBLEM, you need to SOLVE THE PROBLEM.
SOLVING A PROBLEM means FINDING AN ANSWER TO THE PROBLEM.
SOLVING A PROBLEM means MAKING THE PROBLEM GO AWAY.
SOLVING A PROBLEM means FINDING A SOLUTION TO THE PROBLEM.

When you have a PROBLEM, you need to THINK OF WAYS TO MAKE THE PROBLEM GO AWAY.
Here are some WAYS TO MAKE PROBLEMS GO AWAY.
Here are some SOLUTIONS to some PROBLEMS.

> PROBLEM: Not talking to Mom and Dad about things.
>> TROUBLE IT CAUSES: It makes Mom and Dad sad.
> SOLUTION: Talk to Mom and Dad every day.
>> Tell them what you did at school every day.

> PROBLEM: Singing too loudly in a restaurant.
>> TROUBLE IT CAUSES: You bother people in the restaurant.
> SOLUTION: Don't sing in the restaurant. Talk with people instead.

> PROBLEM: Not listening in class.
>> TROUBLE IT CAUSES: Your teacher gets mad at you.
> SOLUTION: Pay attention and listen in class.

When you have a PROBLEM, you need to DO THESE THINGS:
> *THINK ABOUT WHAT THE PROBLEM IS.*
> *THINK ABOUT THE TROUBLE IT CAUSES.*
> *THINK OF A WAY TO MAKE THE PROBLEM GO AWAY.*
> *DO SOMETHING TO MAKE THE PROBLEM GO AWAY.*

WHEN YOU SOLVE A PROBLEM, YOU GET OUT OF TROUBLE.
KNOWING HOW TO SOLVE A PROBLEM IS IMPORTANT.

Problem - Solutions Equations

The therapist should have the child go over the equation verbally many times. The child should be saying something like, "If something is a problem, it will cause trouble". The child should also be given some of the problem/solution situations that are listed on the script to "plug" into this format. This will probably require prompting for a while, but it may be the quickest way to get the child to understand problem/solution by comparing these situations to each other. An additional goal is for the child to learn that these situations illustrate a cause/effect relationship.

Problem - Solutions Equations

Problem = Causes Trouble

SOLUTION =	FINDING AN ANSWER TO A PROBLEM	=	THINKING OF WAYS TO MAKE A PROBLEM GO AWAY	=	SOLVING A PROBLEM	=	GETS YOU OUT OF TROUBLE

Identifying If There is a Problem

This exercise works on the child's ability to identify problems and solutions. Once the child has completed this exercise with prompting, the therapist should fade out the prompts. Eventually the exercise sheet should be faded and the child should do this exercise orally. As the child becomes more familiar with this drill, the parents should use this same structure to point out problems in the child's natural environment and have the child come up with solutions and do them. *Note: It is important to relate "problem" to danger and "no problem" to being safe (wherever appropriate); however, the child must learn that danger is always a problem, but problems do not always refer to danger. This concept is a difficult one that, over time, the child can be taught.*

Identifying If There is a Problem

Read each sentence. If the sentence is talking about a problem, write "problem" on the line. If there is no problem, write "no problem".

Situation	Problem or No Problem?
Not talking to mom and dad. Why? (Prompt) because not talking to Mom and Dad makes them sad.	Problem
Not doing you work. Why? (Prompt) because not doing my work makes my teacher mad.	Problem
Playing with dolls. Why? (Prompt) because playing with dolls is safe.	No Problem
Running in the street.	Problem
Reading a book. Why? (Prompt) because reading a book is _____.	No Problem

Deciding Who to Listen To

The "Deciding Who To Listen To" script should be introduced to work on the child's critical thinking skills. The child and the therapist should alternate reading lines in the script. This script should be read with the child every day for a week or two (until s/he knows the script well). During this time, the child should be asked questions about whom they have to listen to and whom they do not have to listen to. In addition, the child should be given simple situations in which s/he must decide to listen or not.

Deciding Who To Listen To

There are lots of people I should listen to.

When my mom tells me to do something, I should do it.
When my dad tells me to do something, I should do it.
When my grandma tells me to do something, I should do it.
When my teachers tells me to do something, I should do it.
When Shelley or Lorelei or Casey or Sharon tells me to do something, I should do it.

I should always listen to my mom and dad, my grandma, my teachers, and Shelley, Lorelei, Casey, or Sharon.

There are some people that I do not always have to listen to.

When Stacey or Carly tell me to do something, I do not always have to do it.
When Andy and John tell me to do something, I do not always have to do it.
When Josh or Jason or David tell me to do something, I do not always have to do it.
When other kids tell me to do something, I do not always have to do it.
When strangers or people I do not know tell me to do something, I do not always have to do it.

I do not always have to listen to these people.
Before I do what they tell me to do, I need to do these things:

First I need to STOP AND THINK about what I was told to do,
Then I need to ASK MYSELF SOME QUESTIONS,
Last I need to THINK AND DECIDE WHAT TO DO.

Deciding What To Do

This exercise works on the child's critical thinking skills. The drill teaches the child how to weigh various situations and makes the thinking process explicit. The objective is that this technique will be internalized eventually; however, this may take a long time for most children and some children may always have some trouble with critical thought.

Deciding What To Do

Stacey tells me to run across the street.

First, STOP AND THINK

What was I asked to do? to run across the street

Next, ASK MYSELF SOME QUESTIONS

Questions	Answers
Is it safe?	No, It's dangerous
Is it a problem?	Yes. It's a problem
Will I get in trouble?	Yes, I will get in trouble

Then, THINK AND DECIDE WHAT TO DO

What I know: It's dangerous, It's a problem. I will get in trouble..

Decide what to do: I do not run across the street.

I tell Stacey, "I will not run across the street".

How To Teach Advanced Problem/Solutions

The scripts and exercises in the following section are quite advanced and should be reserved for the time when the child has mastered the easier critical thinking exercises. The first exercise is a more advanced version of the Problems/Solution exercise in the preceding section.

First, the therapist should use problems directly from the Problem/Solution Script (since the child should know the script quite well). The list of problems specific to the child should be used, varying the problems in as many ways as possible. For example, if the child has a tendency to sing in restaurants, then the name of the restaurant should be varied so the problem is presented in a slightly different way each time. In addition, by changing the name of the restaurant each time, the child learns to generalize "no singing" to all restaurants rather than just one.

In the beginning, the therapist should read the problem to the child. The child should reply by reading from the Problem/Solutions sheet (immediately following). After the child understands the drill, then the therapist should write the question down and read it back to the child. S/he should then be able to answer without reading the sheet. Eventually the therapist should be able to ask the child verbally, without the child seeing the sheet, and the child should be able to answer.

At first, any reasonable solution the child gives should be accepted. The question probes are important to ensure that the child understands what he reads and is not simply memorizing the answers. This sheet should be done daily until the child understands the problem and its consequences. The therapist should always re-do any "missed" problems until the child learns that specific problem/solution relationship.

It is important to customize all the drills to the child. For example, if the children in the neighborhood are ridiculing others in a particular way, the therapist should write the exact expressions used by the neighborhood children so the child can identify the way children are made fun of in his/her environment.

Once the child can complete the Problem/Solutions exercise, it is time to introduce the "Problem Situations" script. Once the child understands this script, then it is time to introduce "Identifying Trouble and Generating Solutions". The therapist should do this drill with the child for the first few times, attempting to fade out the prompts as soon as the child seems to understand. The idea in this exercise is to teach the child to explicitly go through the evaluation process of a situation. The goal is for the child to eventually internalize the thought process thereby applying it to real-life situations.

The "Being Made Fun Of" script and equation are designed for the child who does not understand the social rules but **does** want to interact with his/her peers. Unfortunately, children can be mean; therefore, the script, equation, and exercises are designed to give the child an understanding of that sort of interaction. The "Identifying If Someone is Being Made Fun Of" exercise should be introduced before the "Identifying If Something

Said is Nice Or Mean" exercise. These concepts can be difficult for children with pervasive developmental disorders and may take a long time to grasp.

The "What To Do When Someone Hurts Me" script is designed to teach the child what to do in a variety of situations when s/he is hurt. The script should be presented several times to the child as explained above.

Why Teach Advanced Problem/Solutions?

This area of critical thinking is full of subtleties; however, the child is going to confront these situations throughout his or her life. It is our goal to prepare the child as much as possible for these socially unfortunate situations in order for the child to better understand the unwritten rules of interpersonal relations. The scripts which address "being made fun of" and "being mean" are two examples of situations that the child should be aware of and should be given the tools to use in order to cope with the situation.

Problem/Solutions

This exercise introduces problems and their solutions. It sets up a formal structure that the child should learn to better understand social rules. To help the child understand this drill, it is very important to customize the examples to situations that arise in the child's life where s/he breaks rules that are often taken for granted as being common sense. The more relevant and realistic the situations, the faster the child will come to understand the concept. This exercise will have to be heavily prompted by the therapist at first; however, once the child understands the drill, the therapist should fade the prompts.

Problem/Solutions

Problem: You are singing to loudly in the restaurant. What should you do?

Solution: (Prompt) I should not sing in the restaurant.

Question probes: Why don't you sing in the restaurant? (Prompt) because it bothers people or it makes people mad.
What should you do in the restaurant? (Prompt) talk with people/or eat my food.

Problem: Your friend tells you to run in the street. What should you do?

Solution: (Prompt) I should not run in the street.

Question probes: Why don't you run in the street? (Prompt) It is dangerous.
What could happen? (Prompt) I could get hit by a car.

Problem: You are not listening in class. What should you do?

Solution: (Prompt) I should listen in class.

Question probes: Who gets mad if you don't listen? (Prompt) My teacher gets mad.
What else happens if you don't listen? (Prompt) I don't know what to do and I get in trouble.

Problem Situations (Target: Dangerous Things)

This script should be read many times, alternating lines between the therapist and child. Then the therapist should ask if these various activities are dangerous and if so, what could happen. The therapist should intersperse non-problems in the questions in order to make sure the child is listening and thinking.

Problem Situations (Target: Dangerous Things)

SITUATION	DANGEROUS EFFECT
RUNNING IN THE STREET is dangerous.	It is a **PROBLEM** because **YOU COULD GET HIT BY A CAR.**
RUNNING IN THE PARKING LOT is dangerous.	It is a **PROBLEM** because **YOU COULD GET HIT BY A CAR.**
JUMPING OFF HIGH THINGS is dangerous.	It is a **PROBLEM** because **YOU COULD GET HURT.**
WALKING AWAY FROM MOM AT THE STORE is dangerous.	It is a **PROBLEM** because **YOU COULD GET LOST.**
GETTING TOO CLOSE TO A FIRE is dangerous.	It is a **PROBLEM** because **YOU COULD GET BURNED.**
PLAYING WITH MATCHES is dangerous.	It is a **PROBLEM** because **YOU COULD GET BURNED.**
NOT WEARING YOUR SEAT BELT is dangerous.	It is a **PROBLEM** because **YOU COULD GET HURT IF YOU GOT IN A CAR ACCIDENT.**
RIDING YOUR BIKE WITHOUT A HELMET ON is dangerous.	It is a **PROBLEM** because **YOU COULD HURT YOUR HEAD IF YOU FELL OFF YOUR BIKE.**
EATING THINGS THAT ARE NOT FOOD is dangerous.	It is a **PROBLEM** because **YOU COULD GET SICK.**
CHEWING ON WIRES OR CORDS is dangerous.	It is a **PROBLEM** because **YOU COULD GET HURT.**

Identifying "Trouble" and Generating Solutions

This exercise structures a critical thinking process that the child should learn in order to understand social rules. It may take a very long time for the child to do this on his/her own. The goal is for the child to eventually generalize this form of critical thinking to his/her natural environment. In order for the child to understand this drill, it is very important to customize examples of situations that arise in the child's life where s/he breaks rules that we take for granted as being common sense. The more relevant and realistic the situations, the faster the child will come to understand this exercise.

Identifying "Trouble" and Generating Solutions

Read each problem. Tell what "trouble" each problem causes. Then give a solution to the problem.

Situation	Trouble the Problem Causes
If: _You are standing in John's_	Then: _John gets mad_
way when he is trying to watch TV	_____

So, Solution: _So I don't stand in John's way_

Situation	Trouble the Problem Causes
If: _You don't have enough money_	Then: _Prompt: (What can't you do?)_
to buy lunch at school	_I can't buy lunch at school_

So, Solution: _I need to get more money_

Being Made Fun Of

The Being Made Fun Of script should be introduced to work on the child's social awareness skills. The child and the therapist should alternate reading lines in the script. This script should be read with the child every day for a week or two (until the child knows the script well). During this time, the child should be asked questions where s/he decides whether the child is being made fun of or whether the children are playing nicely. In addition, it is important for the child to be able to critically evaluate whether s/he is being instructed to do something wrong.

Being Made Fun Of

When kids CALL YOU MEAN NAMES AND LAUGH AT YOU,
they are MAKING FUN OF YOU.
They are TEASING YOU IN A MEAN WAY.

BEING MADE FUN OF IS NOT FUN.
BEING MADE FUN OF IS NOT NICE. It is MEAN.

When you are BEING MADE FUN OF, it HURTS YOUR FEELINGS.
When you GET TEASED IN A MEAN WAY, it MAKES YOU SAD.

These are some MEAN THINGS kids might say to MAKE FUN OF YOU.
     "Hey STUPID, don't you know anything?"
     "You're SO FAT. You're a pig."
     "That's a GROSS haircut. Your hair looks stupid."
     "You're CLUMSY. I don't want to dance with you.
     "You have UGLY clothes on. Those are ugly shoes, too."
     "You STINK. We're not going to play with you."

These are some BAD THINGS kids get you to do to MAKE FUN OF YOU
 AND MAKE YOU LOOK SILLY:
They will always MAKE YOU BE "IT" WHEN YOU PLAY TAG.
They will LAUGH and RUN AWAY FROM YOU.
They might say:
"GRAB Jason and KISS him."
"Go KICK Stacey."
"LOCK David in the bathroom. Don't let him out."
"TAKE Erin's Barbie. Don't let her know where it is."

When someone is MAKING FUN OF YOU, DO NOT LISTEN TO THEM.
When someone is MAKING FUN OF YOU, you can DO THESE THINGS:
You can say, "YOU'RE BEING MEAN. THAT'S NOT COOL." OR
You can WALK AWAY FROM THEM.

BEING MADE FUN OF IS NOT FUN.
BEING TEASED IN A MEAN WAY HURTS YOUR FEELINGS.

NEVER MAKE FUN OF ANYONE.
MAKING FUN OF SOMEONE IS NOT NICE.

Being Made Fun of Equation

The therapist should have the child read the equation aloud many times. The child should be saying something like, "Being made fun of is mean teasing". The child should also be given some of the situations from the script to "plug" into this format. This will probably require prompting for a while, but it may be the quickest way to get the child to understand the equation.

Being Made Fun of Equation

BEING MADE = MEAN TEASING = NOT NICE = HURTS = MAKES YOU SAD
FUN OF   YOUR
                                              FEELINGS

MAKING FUN = TEASING IN A = NOT NICE = DO NOT DO IT
OF SOMEONE   MEAN WAY

Identifying If Someone is Being Made Fun Of

This exercise structures a critical thinking process that the child should learn in order to understand the social interaction of his/her peers. The goal is for the child to be able to recognize when this occurs in his/her natural environment. In order for the child to understand this drill, it is very important to customize situations that arise in the child's life where someone is made fun of. The more relevant and realistic the situations, the faster the child will come to understand this exercise.

Identifying If Someone is Being Made Fun Of

Read about each situation. If the situation shows someone being made fun of or being teased in a mean way, write "being made fun of" or "mean teasing" on the line. If it does not show someone being made fun of, write "not being made fun of" or "no teasing" on the line.

Situation	Being Made Fun of or Not Being Made Fun of?
David is playing tag with Josh and David says, "Josh, you're sooo fat, you couldn't catch a turtle."	being made fun of
Jenny says, "Suzie's so stupid. She's such a retard."	being made fun of
Carla says, "Jenny can't reach the bars. We should help her."	not being made fun of

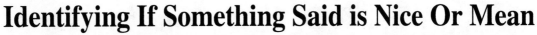

Identifying If Something Said is Nice Or Mean

This exercise teaches the child to judge whether the person s/he is speaking to is being nice or mean. This is important because children with developmental and/or language delays often cannot discern attempts at friendship from teasing. This should be customized to the child so that experiences from the child's environment are reflected in this exercise. This exercise familiarizes the child with common words that are used by children to ridicule others. Aside from particular words that are mean or nice, voice inflection also determines whether something said is nice or mean. This drill should be done at first without mean or nice voice inflection. Once the child learns to identify nice from mean in terms of content, then the drill must be done using the same phrases but varying the voice inflection. Eventually, the child should be taught that mean voice inflection is insulting even if the content is not necessarily bad. For example, the phrase, "I like your hair band" is mean when someone says it in a mean way.

Identifying If Something Said is Nice Or Mean

Read each sentence that is "said". Write down if it is a "nice" thing to say or a "mean" thing to say. Then tell if you can "say" it or if you "don't say" it.

WHAT IS SAID	NICE or MEAN?	SAY or DON'T SAY?
I like your haircut.	Nice	Say
That's a dumb shirt.	Mean	Don't Say
You stink so get lost.	Mean	Don't Say
What a baby you are.	Mean	Don't Say
I like your hair band.	Nice	Say

What To Do When Someone Hurts Me

The What To Do When Someone Hurts Me script should be introduced to work on the child's independence skills. The child and the therapist should alternate reading lines in the script. This script should be read with the child every day for a week or two (until the child knows the script well). During this time, the child should be asked questions about what to do when s/he is hurt.

This
paragraph
must be
customized to
the child!

What To Do When Someone Hurts Me

Sometimes kids will hurt me when I am trying to play near them.
Some kids may try to KICK ME, or HIT ME, or PUSH ME down, or
THROW SOMETHING AT ME.
When someone hurts me, I NEED TO TELL a grown-up person WHO hit me and
WHAT HAPPENED.

If someone HURTS ME when I am AT SCHOOL, I NEED TO FIND A TEACHER.
I need to tell the teacher WHO hurt me.
If I don't know the kid's name, I need to POINT TO THE KID who hurt me.
I need to tell the teacher WHAT HAPPENED.
If a kid hits me, I need to say, "That kid hit me."
If a kid kicks me, I need to say, "That kid kicked me."
If a kid pushes me down, I need to say, "That kid pushed me down."
If a kid throws a rock at me, I need to say, "That kid threw a rock at me."

If someone HURTS ME when I am PLAYING SOCCER AT THE
COMMUNITY CENTER, I NEED TO FIND THE COACH.
I need to tell the coach WHO hurt me.
I need to POINT TO THE KID who hurt me.
I need to tell the coach WHAT HAPPENED.
If a kid kicks me at soccer, I need to say, "That kid kicked me."
If a kid pushes me down, I need to say, "That kid pushed me down."

If someone HURTS ME when I am playing AT THE PARK,
I NEED TO FIND THE PERSON I WENT TO THE PARK WITH.
I need to tell mom or dad or Sue or Debbie or Dave or John WHO hurt me.
I need to POINT TO THE KID who hurt me.
I need to tell mom or dad or Sue or Debbie or Dave or John WHAT HAPPENED.
If a kid pushes me off the slide, I need to say, "That kid pushed me off the slide."
If a kid throws sand in my eyes, I need to say, "That kid threw sand at me."

WHENEVER A PERSON HURTS ME, I NEED TO TELL SOMEONE ABOUT IT.
If is important to let someone know WHO hurt me and WHAT HAPPENED.
I SHOULD ALWAYS TELL SOMEBODY WHEN SOMEONE HURTS ME.

How To Teach Daily Language Requirements

The following scripts should be taught in much the same way as the other scripts introduced in this book. The child and therapist should read through the script alternating lines. Once the child has read through the script many times and knows the script well, either the therapist or child should write down each step on a separate piece of paper and then have the child put the slips of paper in the correct sequence.

This should be done as follows:

1. The therapist writes each component or step on a separate slip of paper.
2. The therapist mixes up the slips of paper.
3. The therapist instructs the child to put the slips of paper in the correct sequence to ensure that the child comprehends the steps.

Once the child has sequenced the steps, then the child and the therapist should act out the script. For the ordering food script, the therapist should be the cashier. Once this verbal exchange is relatively easy for the child, then the child should go to a fast food restaurant and order food. Once the child is comfortable doing this, s/he should order food whenever the opportunity arises. The idea is for the child to become comfortable with this verbal exchange and be able to use this skill in a variety of ordering situations.

In every situation where the child is required to look after his or her own interests, a script should be written and taught to him/her. The script must be customized to the specific situation for it to be of maximum value for the child.

Why Teach Daily Language Requirements?

High level self help skills are generally language based and must be taught if the child is to be independent. Ordering food and answering the telephone are simply two language based examples of this; however, there are countless others that can be taught in the same manner. Any language-based requirements that the child has should be customized to that child, whether it is something as simple as the "Trick or Treat" verbal exchange of a young child or a job based verbal requirement of an adult. If there is a verbal structure, it should be made explicit and taught. The child will internalize the structure and have a much easier time during each verbal exchange.

Ordering My Food

The Ordering My Food script should be introduced to work on the child's independence skills. The child and the therapist should alternate reading lines in the script. This script should be read with the child every day for a week or two (until the child knows the script well). During this time, the child should be asked questions about the sequence of ordering food. In this way, s/he will learn the routine and know what is expected. Once the child learns the script, s/he should be taken to a fast food restaurant and follow the steps sequenced in the script.

Ordering My Food

When I go to McDonald's, Burger King, or any other fast food place, **I NEED TO DO THESE THINGS.**

I GET IN LINE.
> I pay attention and move forward in line.
> When I get to the front of the line, I walk to the counter.

I TELL THE CASHIER WHAT I WANT TO EAT.
> I say, "I would like a _____, _____, and _____."
> I pay attention and answer the cashier's questions.
> If the cashier asks, "Do you want a large, medium, or small drink?", I tell the cashier what I want.
> If the cashier asks, "Do you want cheese on your hamburger?", I tell the cashier what I want.
> If the cashier asks, "Do you want any ketchup?", I tell her "yes, please" if I want some ketchup.
> If the cashier says, "For here or to go?", I say:
>> "for here" if I want to eat my food at McD's or Burger King,
>> or
>> "to go" if I want to take my food home to eat.

I WAIT UNTIL THE CASHIER TELLS ME HOW MUCH MONEY I NEED TO GIVE HER FOR MY FOOD.
> I give the cashier my money.
> I wait for my change.
> I put the change in my pocket.

I WAIT FOR MY FOOD.
> Sometimes I am given an order number.
> The cashier gives me a piece of paper with my food order number and might say, "You're order number 36."
> I need to look at my piece of paper and listen for my order number to be called.
> When my number is called, I pick up my tray or bag of food.

I GET A NAPKIN AND A STRAW FROM THE COUNTER.
If I am eating at McDonald's or Burger King, I FIND A CLEAN TABLE, SIT DOWN, AND EAT MY FOOD.
WHEN I AM FINISHED EATING, I THROW AWAY MY GARBAGE.

Answering the Telephone

The Answering the Telephone script helps the child sequence the events of the interaction. Talking on the telephone is very difficult for people with language delays and the script helps the child practice. The Answering the Telephone script should be copied onto Card Stock, put up by the telephone and customized to the child.

Answering the Phone

1. **PICK UP** the phone. Put it to your ear and mouth.

2. **SAY,** "Hello. This is Sue."

3. **WAIT** for the caller to say something.

4. **ASK,** "Who is calling?"

5. **WAIT** for the caller to say their name.

6. **ASK,** "Who do you want to talk to?"

7. **WAIT** for the caller to say who they want.

8. **SAY,** "Here _____ this is for you. It's _____."

9. **GIVE** the phone to the person the caller wants to talk to.

How To Teach Fact or Opinion

Prerequisite: This is a high level activity and should not be taught until the child has completed and mastered the more basic language drills at the beginning of every chapter.

1. The therapist must first describe the difference between fact and opinion by saying:
   "A FACT IS A SENTENCE THAT IS TRUE ABOUT SOMETHING".
   "AN OPINION IS SOMETHING THAT A PERSON THINKS".

2. Then the therapist should use the opinion phrases on the following three pages to have a conversation with the child. The therapist and child should take turns choosing a card from the pile and turning it over once the opinion statement has been made.

3. Once the child is comfortable with using the opinion phrases, then the therapist should introduce the Multiple Opinion sheet and choose a topic that the child is interested in e.g. food, movies, sports, animals. This sheet should be used many times (until the therapist is certain that the child understands the drill well).

4. The next step is to use the "Opinions and Supporting Reasons: Food" sheet. The introduction of a supporting reason may be difficult at first for the child to understand; however, it is important because that is going to help internalize the concept of opinion. This sheet can be used for other topics once it has been customized.

5. The Fact or Opinion sheet is the next activity to introduce. Introducing facts and opinion at the same time should be relatively easy for the child to grasp. If it is not, then the first four steps were covered too quickly and should be revisited until the child is ready for this stage. The fact or opinion sheet should be customized to many topics relevant to the child. Examples of topics other than food have been included (e.g. movies, sports) to give the therapist an idea of how to customize the sheet to the child and the situation.

When doing the five drills described above, it is important to emphasize to the child that these are all opinions.

 # Why Teach Fact Or Opinion?

It is very important that the child be able to differentiate between fact and opinion since the child must learn to critically evaluate information when it is presented. In addition, much conversation is about people exchanging opinions. The child must know that an opinion does not have to be acted upon or agreed with in order to be exchanged.

Cards To Teach Fact or Opinion

These are reproducible cards to be used as explained on the previous page. They can be photocopied onto card stock to ensure their durability.

Opinion Phrases	**I believe**
In my opinion	**My favorite**
I like	**I don't like**
I think the best	**I don't think**

Cards For Teaching Fact or Opinion

These are reproducible game cards to be used as explained on the previous page. They can be photocopied onto card stock to ensure their durability.

I feel	**I Think**
Questions you can ask to find out about other people's opinions	**Opinion Questions**
How do you feel about...?	**What do you think about...?**
What's your opinion about...?	**Do you believe that...?**

Cards For Teaching Fact or Opinion

These are reproducible game cards to be used as explained on the previous page. They can be photocopied onto card stock to ensure their durability.

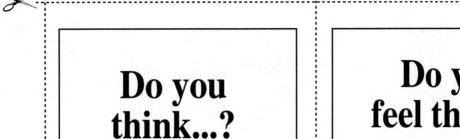

Do you think...?

Do you feel that...?

Multiple Opinions

This drill has the child formulate and express opinions on one particular topic. Food is a good topic to begin with since most children have opinions about food. This sheet uses several different ways to convey the same negative or positive opinions. It is important for the child to know these different words so that they can understand them when other children and adults use them.

Multiple Opinions

My opinions about: _____ food _____

My favorite ___ food is ice-cream sandwiches. ___

I like ___ candy. ___

I don't like ___ broccoli. ___

I believe that ___ corn tastes good. ___

I think the best ___ candy is chocolate. ___

I feel that ___ cake is a good dessert. ___

I think that ___ chips taste salty. ___

I don't think that ___ peas taste good. ___

In my opinion ___ jello is fun. ___

I can't stand ___ mustard. ___

One of the worst ___ foods is lettuce. ___

Opinions and Supporting Reasons: Food

The following exercise gives the child a structure within which to voice an opinion and sets up a set of reasons from which to choose. It is important to make sure the topics chosen are familiar to the child and that the child has an opinion about them. Food is a particularly good topic since children have definite preferences in this area.

Opinions and Supporting Reasons: Food

Choose 3 _____ foods _____ :

Food	Opinion	Supporting Reason

cheerios

(like) don't like   (good)   sour   crunchy
delicious   awful   gooey
juicy   bad   cold
sweet   too spicy   hot

I like cheerios because they're good.

oatmeal

like (don't like)   good   sour   crunchy
delicious   awful   gooey
juicy   bad   cold
sweet   too spicy (hot)

I don't like oat meal because it's hot.

bagels

(like) don't like   good   sour   crunchy
(delicious) awful   gooey
juicy   bad   cold
sweet   too spicy   hot

I like bagels because they're delicious.

I like toast and butter because it tastes good.

Opinions and Supporting Reasons: Movies

This exercise gives the child a structure within which to voice an opinion and provides a set of reasons from which to choose. It is important to make sure the topics chosen are familiar to the child and that the child has an opinion about them. The topic, "Movies" is more difficult than food, but is a good topic since most typically developing children have opinions about movies.

Opinions and Supporting Reasons: Movies

Choose 3 _____ movies _____:

Movies	Opinion	Supporting Reason

Lion King

I like The Lion King because it's scary.

Opinion: (like)   don't like

Supporting Reason:
boring   exciting
(scary)   funny
bad   good
too hard to   entertaining
understand   (fun to watch)

Pocahontas

I like Pocahontas because it's exciting.

Opinion: (like)   don't like

Supporting Reason:
boring   (exciting)
scary   funny
bad   good
too hard to   entertaining
understand   (fun to watch)

Jurassic Park

I don't like Jurassic Park because it's too hard to understand.

Opinion: like   (don't like)

Supporting Reason:
boring   exciting
scary   funny
bad   good
(too hard to   entertaining
understand)   (fun to watch)

I like cartoon movies because they are fun to watch.

Fact Or Opinion?

This exercise teaches a child the difference between a person's opinion and a factual statement. The topic should interest the child and be a topic the child knows something about. The first part of the exercise has the child distinguish between opinion and fact; the second part gives the child the opportunity to tell the therapist a fact about the topic and give his/her opinion about the topic. The category of foods is a good category to begin with since many children have opinions about food.

Fact Or Opinion?

Read each statement about the topic or event. Tell whether it is a fact or an opinion. Then state one more fact about the topic/event and give your own opinion about the topic/event.

Topic or Event: ___Food___   Fact or Opinion?

Apples are my favorite fruit.   Opinion

Apples are good for you.   Fact

Chocolate is sweet.   Fact

I can't stand chocolate.   Opinion

Fact about: ____food____   Watermelon is fruit.

_____

My Opinion about: ___food___   Watermelon is my
favorite fruit.

possible prompts are:
I think,
I like,
I feel,
I believe,
My favorite

Fact Or Opinion? (Movies)

This exercise teaches a child the difference between a person's opinion and a factual statement. The topic should interest the child and be a topic the child knows something about. The first part of the exercise has the child differentiate between opinion and fact, the second part gives the child the opportunity to tell the therapist a fact about the topic and give his/her opinion about it. The category of movies the child enjoys is an example of a good topic to choose, even if s/he does not fully understand the movie.

Fact Or Opinion?

Read each statement about the topic or event. Tell whether it is a fact or an opinion. Then state one more fact about the topic/event and give your own opinion about the topic/event.

Topic or Event: _The Lion King movie_ **Fact or Opinion?**

The Lion King is about Simba and Nala — _Fact_

I don't like Scar because he's mean — _Opinion_

My favorite character was Pumba — _Opinion_

The lions lived on Pride Rock — _Fact_

Fact about: _The Lion King_ — The Lion King is about lions in Africa.

My Opinion about: _The Lion King_ — I think that the Lion King is a sad movie.

possible prompts are:
I think,
I like,
I feel,
I believe,
My favorite

Fact Or Opinion?

This exercise is a variant of the preceding exercise. It teaches a child the difference between a person's opinion and a factual statement. The topic should interest the child and be a topic that the child knows something about. The first part of the exercise has the child discern between opinion and fact, the second part gives the child the opportunity to tell the therapist a fact about the topic and give his/her opinion about the topic. The Academy of Sciences is an example of a topic that is more advanced than food, but would be relevant to the child if s/he had just visited the museum.

Fact Or Opinion?

Read each statement about the topic or event. Tell whether it is a fact or an opinion. Then state one more fact about the topic/event and give your own opinion about the topic/event.

Topic or Event: _Academy of Sciences_   Fact or Opinion?

The Academy of Sciences is in San Francisco	Fact
My favorite place to go to is the Academy of Sciences	Opinion
I like seeing the dinosaurs at the Academy of Sciences	Opinion
The Academy of Sciences has different things to see.	Fact

Fact about: _Academy of Sciences_   The Academy of Sciences has animals.

My Opinion about: _Academy of Sciences_   I think I don't like the food at the Academy of Sciences.

possible prompts are:
I think,
I like,
I feel,
I believe,
My favorite

My Opinions (About School)

This exercise is designed to show the child the difference between opinions and facts by having the child list his/her opinions above a list of facts about his/her school. Once the child lists his/her opinions, then the child should read through the facts about the school. The therapist should then read an opinion or a fact and ask the child to identify what the statement is i.e. fact or opinion.

My Opinions (About School)

My Opinions About School

In school the thing I like to do best is ___math___.

My favorite thing to do at recess is ___playing on the bars.___

At school I don't like to ___do reading___

When they have ___carrots___ for lunch I don't like to eat it.

I think that school is ___fun___.

Facts about my school:

The name of my school is Belmont Elementary.

Lots of kids go to my school.

There is hot lunch at my school.

The playground at school is large.

There are many classrooms at my school.

My Opinions (Movies)

This exercise is designed to show the child the difference between opinions and facts by having the child list his/her opinions above a list of facts about movies. Once the child lists his/her opinions, then the child should read through the facts about movies. The therapist should then read an opinion or a fact and ask the child to identify what the statement is i.e. fact or opinion.

My Opinions (Movies)

My Opinions About Movies

My favorite movie is ___Pocahontas___. I like it because ___I like the songs.___

The scariest movie I have ever seen is ___Bambi___.

The funniest movie I have ever seen is ___Jungle book___.

I don't like ___Bambi___ because ___of the hunter___.

___101 Dalmatians___ is a good movie.

Facts about movies:

Movies are about people, places, and things.

You can see movies at the movie theater.

> The Lion King is about Simba and Nala.
> Pocahontas is about Pocahontas and John Smith.
> Snow White is about Snow White and the Seven Dwarfs.
> Beauty and the Beast is about Belle and the Beast.

3 General Knowledge

Increasing General Knowledge

Introducing and Maintaining Information
- Topic One: Animals
- Scripts, Exercises, and Samples
- Topic Two: Occupations/Community Helpers
- Scripts, Exercises, and Samples
- Topic Three: Places in the Community
- Scripts, and Samples
- Topic Four: Sports
- Scripts, Exercises, and Samples
- Other Topics

Creating Information Paragraphs

Comparisons
- Exercises

Concluding Remarks About General Knowledge

What's Next In Terms of General Information?

How To Use This Chapter

The exercises in this chapter are introduced using the first two topics that the child should learn: animals and occupations. The activities are introduced with an explanation and rationale for each drill. These drills should be adapted to a variety of subjects (ideas of other topics are given following the animal and occupation sections). Once the child learns the structure of each exercise, s/he can use the exercises to organize new material introduced to him/her in school or through books. It will become obvious to the therapist or parent how easily the drills can be adapted to any subject.

In order to become familiarized with the drills before introducing them to the child, the therapist should read all the information given about animals, including examples of the drills provided. Once the child has learned about animals based on the paragraphs and drills provided, s/he is ready to learn about professions. The therapist should then read all the information and drills provided on professions before beginning this next topic with the child. Most of the activities used with animals have been applied to professions. The reason we have included these drills (in spite of the apparent repetition) is to enable the therapist to see how to adapt these drills to other topics not included in this book.

It is useful to expand upon the topics provided here with age appropriate videotapes, books and computer games. Below is a very basic list of materials that have been helpful in creating new topics and promoting general knowledge (to be used by the parent or child depending upon level of difficulty):

BOOKS

The Eye Opener Series, A Dorling Kindersley Book, Published by Aladdin Books, a publishing division of Simon and Schuster, 1991.

Rockie Read About Science Series, Children's Press, Chicago, 1992.

Scholastic First Discovery Book Series, Cartwheel Books, Scholastic, Inc. My First Book Of Facts.

"I can be a" series on professions, published by Children's Press, Chicago, Regensteiner Publishing Enterprises, Inc.

Scholastic First series: 1) Encyclopedia; 2) Animals and Nature; 3) How Things Work, published by Scholastic Inc., 1995.

Increasing General Knowledge

Most children with autism spectrum disorders are visual learners. Using the visual channel to teach these children gives them more opportunity to absorb information missed auditorially.

An additional tool used to introduce general information to children with pervasive developmental disorders is to give a structure with which to organize great amounts of information. This is very important! Regardless of topic, ability to use structure is a major strength of children with language disorders. Since these children thrive on structure, introducing structured information gives them the opportunity to keep up with, and sometimes surpass, their normally developing peers in terms of knowledge on specific subjects.

The topics covered in this chapter are designed as a starting point for the child. New topics should be adapted to, and taught, using this structured approach. Many children will learn to identify the structure of topics by themselves once they have done enough drills of the kind in this book. Very quickly, parents and therapists will understand how to find the structure in any topic they need to introduce.

The topics covered here are: animals; professions; places in the community; sports; geography; planets; habitats. Once the child has amassed knowledge on a topic from the paragraphs provided, the child can continue to read about the topic from easy books. After learning the critical information about a topic, the child will be able to read more about the topic and, thereby, add new knowledge to his/her existing knowledge base.

NOTE: For an in-depth discussion on the way children with language delays process language, we highly recommend the book: Ellyn Lucas Arwood, Semantic and Pragmatic Language Disorders. Aspen Publishers, 1991.

Why Increase General Knowledge?

This chapter is devoted to increasing the general knowledge of the child with a pervasive developmental disorder because general knowledge is such an important foundation for learning other information. Children who do not pick up information incidentally, miss much of the information that is naturally absorbed by normally developing children from birth. It is unreasonable and unrealistic to expect children with autism to become interested in age-appropriate information when they have a limited foundation upon which to interpret this information. Therefore, it is necessary to teach basic, general information in a way that these children can absorb and become interested in it. This technique provides a "hook" into age-appropriate information that all children are bombarded with every day.

How To Introduce & Maintain Information

Introducing Information

The parent or therapist should sit with the child at a table or on the floor (which ever location the child is used to working at), and read the paragraph slowly, with a fair amount of feeling. If the child can read, then s/he should follow along. If the child cannot read, s/he should still follow the therapist's finger.

Once the paragraph has been read aloud, the therapist or child should read it again. If the child can read, it is a good opportunity to have him/her read it or to alternate reading lines with the therapist. Alternating keeps the child focused because s/he must follow in order to read the line when it is his/her turn. Another option is to do a combination of the above. For example, the therapist reads and stops at CRITICAL information, letting the child read the critical information aloud.

Once the paragraph has been read a second time, the therapist should ask questions regarding the paragraph, and visually prompt the child with the answer by showing the child the place in the text where the answer lies. For example, if the first line reads, "Lions are big cats", the therapist should ask, "What are Lions?", and point to the first line. Each idea in the entire paragraph should be put into question form orally, line by line. Once the child understands that the answer lies in the text, then s/he can be asked questions out of order. The idea is to teach the child that information can be obtained by reading; specifically, answers to factual questions can be found in text. This principle is important since it will teach the child to **comprehend** text, rather than simple decode words. Once the child has mastered this skill (which may occur quickly or slowly, depending upon the age and reading ability of the child), then the therapist should 1) read the paragraph to the child, 2) take the paragraph away, and 3) ask questions without prompting for the answer. In this way, the child must concentrate on understanding information being presented auditorially (a general weakness for most children with pervasive developmental disorders). The goal is for the child to eventually process this information auditorially because the therapist has already given him/her the structure of what is being presented.

High level information is better presented visually, through the child reading the information; however, it is important to work on the auditory processing deficit because most instruction and information is given orally, particularly in mainstream classroom settings.

A considerably more advanced way to use this activity is to teach note taking. Once the child is 8 years old or older, the therapist may introduce the paragraph by reading it together with the child. Then the therapist should read the paragraph again, slowly and with emphasis. The child is required to write down notes about the paragraph, while the therapist reads it, without seeing the paragraph a second time. Eventually, the therapist can read paragraphs and have the child take notes without the child reading through the paragraph the first time. At this point, the child is relying completely on auditory information, rather than visual information. Once s/he is good at reading paragraphs and answering questions, easy note-taking should be taught. Chapter 6 has a section on teaching note-taking.

New Vocabulary From Paragraphs

When the child encounters new vocabulary within a paragraph, it is important to teach the meaning of the word. The child should learn the new vocabulary through seeing an example of the new word. If that is not possible (if the word is too abstract) then the child should be given a description of the new word by pairing it with a word or phrase the child already knows. An example of this is, exhausted = very tired. A more comprehensive way to teach vocabulary is in Chapter 6.

Maintaining Information

In order for the child to retain the information presented thus far, there are four activity work sheets that the child should complete either verbally and/or in written form. There are undoubtedly more activities that can be created, but these activities are a good place to start.
The four activities are:
1. Verb Grid
2. Oral Definitions
3. Topical Outline
4. Fill in the Blanks
Each of these drills is presented in this chapter with a technique and its rationale.

As the child is introduced to more subjects and shows good retention of information, the information attained should be tied into other subjects. For example, once the child learns about enough animals, animals should then be tied into all the various continents and/or animal habitats. In this way, general knowledge about geography can be connected to the knowledge base the child already has - animals. A large map of the world is useful to make geography concepts more concrete.

Why Teach General Knowledge?

In order to work on the child's ability to use language, there must be a basic knowledge foundation upon which language can be practiced. The best information to introduce and maintain is that which has not been absorbed by the child but which the child is expected to know. This introductory knowledge is used as a "springboard" into the world of general knowledge.

Topic One: Animals

The first category of general knowledge used in this chapter is animals. The following pages give examples of paragraphs written at three levels. If the child is a pre-reader, the easiest level should be used. If the child can read, then the therapist should start with the easiest level and progress at the child's pace. There is no reason to introduce material at too low a level for the child since boredom may create compliance problems. On the other hand, beginning at too high a level will cause frustration and should be avoided.

Animal Categories

Easiest: FARM ANIMALS: Chicken, Horse, Cow, Pig
             ZOO ANIMALS: Monkey, Lion

Medium: MISCELLANEOUS: Bears, Snakes, Bees, Penguins
             JUNGLE: Giraffe, Elephant, Tiger

Difficult: GROUPS: Mammals, Reptiles, Amphibians, Birds, Fish, Insects

NOTE: All other popular animals that are not in the easiest, or medium categories are in the hardest category because it is easier for the parent or therapist to simplify the hardest level, than to create the hardest level. Examples of animals in this category in addition to the ones listed above are Grasshoppers, Frogs, and Snakes.

Animal Drills: Do In Order

The exercises must be done in the following order. The idea is to introduce the easier exercises first, followed by the more difficult exercises.

1. Outline For Topical Information
2. Fill-In-The-Blanks
3. Oral Definitions
4. Grid Fill-In
5. True or False
6. Venn Diagram Comparisons
7. A Variety of Advanced Comparisons

Due to their level of difficulty, Drills 6 and 7 are found in the section on General Comparisons at the end of the chapter.

 # Why Teach About Animals?

Animals are not crucial for children to learn; however, we use animals as a starting point for several reasons: 1) all normally developing children learn about animals from toddler hood; 2) these children will be required to have basic knowledge about animals throughout life; 3) animals are a relatively concrete and interesting topic for children, and 4) animals are all around us and, therefore, make relevant material to base language drills on.

How To Create Animal Scripts

When the easiest animal paragraphs have been learned but the child is not ready to advance to the next level, the therapist or parent can go to the medium and harder paragraphs and extract the four **critical** pieces of information that answer the following questions and put them into easy paragraph form:

1. What is a (<u>xxxxx</u>)? An animal, an insect, etc...
2. Where does a (<u>xxxxx</u>) live? In the jungle, at the zoo, in Africa, in Asia etc...
3. What does a (<u>xxxxx</u>) have that is special to that animal? An elephant has a trunk, a zebra has black and white stripes etc...
4. What does a (<u>xxxxx</u>) eat? Leaves and twigs, fruit and insects etc...

When the child exhausts the hardest paragraphs, it is probably time for him/her to graduate to beginner animal **books** that are factually based. Using the structure learned in this chapter, the child should be able to read the paragraphs in easy books on animals (with help) and learn about the animal from the book.

Samples

EASIEST ANIMAL INFORMATION PARAGRAPHS:

Note:
Each animal paragraph must be presented by itself to the child in a large format (8 1/2 by 11 inch sheet of paper).

Zebras

A zebra is a horse. It has black and white stripes. Zebras live in Africa. They eat grass. Some zebras have fat stripes. Some Zebras have skinny stripes.

Lions

Lions are big cats. They live in Africa. Lions are meat-eaters. They eat other animals. Boy lions have long, thick hair on their heads. The thick hair is called a mane.

MEDIUM ANIMAL INFORMATION PARAGRAPHS:

Elephants

Elephants are the biggest animals that live on land. An elephant has big ears, a long trunk, and two white tusks. The tusks are really long teeth. Elephants drink water with their trunks. Elephants live where it is hot. They eat grass, leaves, and fruit.

Giraffes

The giraffe is the tallest animal in the world. It lives in a country called Africa. You can also see a giraffe at a zoo. Giraffes like to eat leaves and twigs. Twigs are small branches from a tree. A giraffe stretches its long neck up into the trees to eat the leaves and twigs.

DIFFICULT ANIMAL INFORMATION PARAGRAPHS:

Note:
Each
animal
paragraph
must be
presented
by itself to
the child in
a large
format (8
1/2 by 11
inch sheet
of paper).

Chimpanzees

A chimpanzee is a kind of ape. It is a monkey-like animal. It is also a mammal. Chimpanzees live in the jungles of Africa. They sleep in nests that they build in trees.

Chimpanzees eat fruits, nuts, leaves and vegetables.

Chimpanzees usually walk on four legs. They do not have tails. Their hair is long and black. But, their face, ears, hands, and feet do not have hair!

Chimpanzees are very smart. They are good toolmakers. They learn to use sticks and rocks to open nuts.

Amphibians

Amphibians are a group of animals. There are many different kinds of amphibians. Frogs, toads, newts, and salamanders are amphibians.

Amphibians have a backbone just like reptiles and mammals. The skin of amphibians is smooth and wet.

Amphibians live in or near water. They eat slugs, insects, and other small things that live in the water.

Amphibians lay eggs.

Mammals

Mammals are a group of animals. There are many different kinds of mammals. People, monkeys, dogs, and elephants are mammals.

Mammals are warm-blooded. They have a backbone. Mammals have hair or fur on their bodies. A baby mammal drinks milk from its mother's body.

Mammals live all over the world. They eat many different things. Some mammals eat meat, and some mammals eat plants. Many mammals eat both meat and plants.

Insects

Insects are the biggest group of animals. There are many different kinds of insects. Grasshoppers, bees, and beetles are all insects.

Insects have six legs. Their bodies have three parts. Most insects have wings. They are usually small.

Insects have skeletons on the outside of their bodies to protect them.

Insects live all over the world.

Insects eat many different things. Some eat plants, and some eat other insects.

How To Introduce Topical Outlines

The topical outlines should be introduced in the following manner:

1. Easy
First, the therapist reads the paragraph that she has chosen for the child. She should have the outline completely written out <u>in full sentences</u>. Then the therapist has the child read about the paragraph from the outline. The child should read the whole sentence.

2. Medium
Once the child understands that the outline relates to the paragraph (after two or three times for some children), then the therapist should read the paragraph that she has chosen for the child and have the outline completed <u>in point form</u>. The child should then use the outline to tell the therapist about the paragraph. S/he should be prompted to use full sentences even though the child is relying on one word to create an entire sentence.

3. Difficult
Using the topical outline sheet, the child reads the paragraph and then dictates what should be on the outline, while the therapist writes down what the child says, only using one key word per line. Then, the therapist should review the outline with the child, requiring him/her to make full sentences from the point form notes the child has dictated.

A typical difficult drill (Step 3) will sound like the following example:
Therapist: "Tell me four things about the animal." *If the paragraph has six details about the animal, the therapist would ask for six "things" about the animal.*
Child: "Africa."
Therapist: "Good. Lions live in Africa."
The therapist prompts the child to say the whole sentence by turning it into a complete sentence for the child - modeling it for the child. The therapist should accept any CRITICAL piece of information the child gives and write it in point form. The child may be able to give only one piece of information unprompted. The therapist will then continue.
Therapist: "What does a Lion eat?"
Child: "Meat."
With prompting, the therapist models the correct sentence to have the child say, "A Lion eats meat". This back and forth continues until four things are written down. Then the therapists asks the child questions about the paragraph.
Therapist: "What's the topic?"
Child (reading the sheet): "Lions."
Therapist: "What's the most important thing about lions?"
Child: "Lions are big cats."
Therapist: "Tell me four things about Lions."
Child (prompted to count on his/her fingers silently with each piece of information given):
"Lions live in Africa."
"Lions eat meat."
"Lions eat other animals."

Topical Outlines Continued...

"Lions have a mane."

Once the child successfully names four characteristics about a lion, the therapist should take the outline away and ask the child the same, exact questions. The child now must rely on his/her auditory channel and memory. Eventually, the child should be able to auditorially process the information and not require a Topical Outline sheet for recall. This is the eventual goal of the drill.

Once the child has gone over the Topical Outline, it is time to introduce the Simple Child-Generated Outline. The sheet is designed for the child to complete by him/herself. The therapist should introduce this sheet in much the same way as she used the Topical Outline. Once the child can complete the Child-Generated Outline easily, then the Child-Generated Outline with Elaborative Statements should be introduced. Eventually, the child should be able to complete the multi-paragraph outline orally (although this is a very advanced skill). Note: With a verbal child, always do the verbal exercise with and without the outline. After the child can talk about the paragraph with the visual prompt (the outline), it is important to always do the exercise using the child's auditory channel only; otherwise, the child will become dependent upon the outline.

The following section explains how to do the Simple Child-Generated outline. When reading the following section, the therapist should refer to the completed outline to gain a better understanding of how to do the exercise with the child.

The next drill (the Simple Outline) has the child tell the therapist about the paragraph without the therapist completing a Topical Outline. The therapist asks the child, "What is the paragraph about?", and then writes down the child's answer under "Topic". Then the therapist says, "Tell me about Monkeys (topic)." The therapist prompts the child to tell her three things and writes them under "details". Then the child uses this outline to verbally tell the therapist about the topic. Once the child has successfully told the therapist about the topic using the outline, the child should tell the therapist about the same topic without using the outline.

Once the child can do this easily, it is time to introduce the "Simple Outline with Elaborative Statement". The therapist and child work with the sheet in the same way as the Simple Outline, but this time the therapist asks for an elaborative statement. For example,
Therapist: "Tell me about Monkeys (topic)."
Child: "live in jungles."
Therapist: "Good. Tell me something about jungles (the detail)."
Child: "Africa."
This constitutes the Elaborative Statement. The child then uses his/her outline to verbally tell the therapist, in full sentences, about the topic. Once the child has successfully told the therapist about the topic using the outline with the elaborative statement, the child should tell the therapist about the topic again without using the outline.

Topical Outlines Continued...

Once the child is comfortable with elaborative statements, the therapist can introduce the Multi-Paragraph Outline. This outline is quite difficult; therefore, it is important to make sure the child has fully grasped elaborative statements and is ready for this advanced exercise. Also, the child must have enough background knowledge about the topic (based on all the paragraphs read prior to this level) to write a multi-paragraph outline. The therapist can begin the drill in the same way as with the easier level outlines, asking for the topic and some information about the topic. Next, she should ask the child to give examples of that topic. The examples may not be included in the paragraph just read. The child must rely on previously obtained knowledge. Each example becomes the main topic of a paragraph. Then, the child is asked to give three details about each paragraph topic. Once the outline is completed, the child uses it to verbally tell the therapist about the topic. The last step is for the child to tell the therapist about the topic without relying on the outline.

Why Teach Topical Outlines

Topical outlines clarify the structure of the paragraph for the child. The goal is for the child to take other paragraphs and organize them in a way that it is easy to understand and memorize. In addition, the topical outline is used as a crutch for those children who have a very difficult time making a complete sentence. The right type of word (e.g. verb or noun) often helps trigger the rest of the sentence. To illustrate, some children have a difficultly finding the correct verb to use. If the child is given only one word per line, but that word is a verb, then the rest of the sentence will be easier for the child to complete. Using outlines to prompt speech also gets the child used to talking, even though the speech is highly structured and patterned.

Outline For Topical Information

This exercise teaches the child 1) how to learn from the written word, and 2) how to distinguish between main idea and detail. To make this drill easy or intermediate, the outline should be completed by the therapist before the session. To make this drill more difficult, the child should fill in the details with the therapist during the drill. First, the child reads the paragraph with the therapist. Then the therapist uses the outline to help the child comprehend and talk about the paragraph.

Outline For Topical Information

Topic: _____ eagles _____

Main Idea: ____ eagles are big birds ____

Details: ____ nests ____

____ long beak ____

____ feathers ____

____ swoops ____

____ trees ____

____ small mammals and birds ____

____ hunt - sky ____

____ talons ____

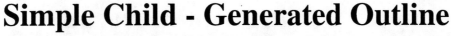

Simple Child - Generated Outline

This exercise teaches the child how to comprehend the written word and differentiate main idea and detail. This outline should be completed by the child during the session after the therapist has gone over the easy and intermediate therapist-generated outline with the child. First the child reads the paragraph. Then the child dictates the information to the therapist. At first, the child should be expected to give one word only. Eventually, the child should be able to tell the therapist about the topic in full sentences by using these single words as prompts. Once the child has mastered this skill, s/he should be given the opportunity to write a short paragraph based on his/her outline. This drill can be introduced once the child is familiar with topical outlines and knows how to write.

Simple Outline For Topical Information

Topic: _eagles_

Tell me about _eagles_ .

Main Idea: _bird_

Details: _nests_

feathers

sky

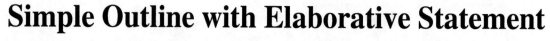

Simple Outline with Elaborative Statement

This outline, like the simple outline, should be completed by the child during the session. First the child should read the paragraph with the therapist. Then the child should dictate the words to be written on the outline to the therapist. The child should give a detail and then elaborate on that detail. Once the child has mastered the Outline with Elaborative Statement, s/he should be given the opportunity to write a short paragraph based on his/her outline.

Outline For Topical Information (Elaborative)

Topic: _eagles_

Tell me about _eagles_

Main Idea: _bird_

big - predator

nests

lays eggs

feathers

warm

sky

swoops prey

Multi-Paragraph Outline

This advanced exercise should be introduced only when the child has a firm grasp of the "Simple Outline with Elaborate Statement". The outline should be completed by the child during the session on topical outlines. After the child reads the paragraph with the therapist, s/he should dictate the relevant information to the therapist. The therapist should ask questions when the child is stuck. The child should give the therapist 1) the topic, and a few details about the topic, and 2) examples of the topic. Those examples become the main idea for the smaller paragraphs. Then, the child should be asked to come up with three details for each secondary topic. Using this completed outline, the child should be able to talk about the topic.

Multi-Paragraph Outline For Topical Information

Topic: _____ Mammals _____

General Info: _____ many kinds _____

_____ warmblooded _____

_____ backbone _____

1. Topic: _____ Lion _____

Details: _____ Africa _____

_____ meat-eaters _____

_____ mane _____

3. Topic: _____ Bear _____

Details: _____ mountains _____

_____ honey _____

_____ sleep in winter _____

2. Topic: _____ Elephant _____

Details: _____ hot _____

_____ grass, leaves, _____

_____ trunk, tusks _____

4. Topic: _____ Kangaroos _____

Details: _____ Australia _____

_____ plants, bushes _____

_____ pouch _____

Animal Fill-In-The-Blanks

After the therapist and child have read a paragraph and completed the easiest topical outline, the therapist should introduce "Animal Fill In The Blanks" exercise. The therapist should read the sentences with blanks to the child and stop at the blank. The child will then be prompted to answer by filling in the blank. Generally, the children remember the paragraph well enough to be able to complete the blanks; therefore, it is important that the "Fill In The Blanks" structure closely resembles the paragraph. This exercise is another tool to use to focus the child's attention on what is important in the paragraph. The "Blanks" can be customized to target the child's weakness. For example, a child who has difficulty with verbs can be required to complete a "Fill-In-The-Blanks" exercise where all the blanks are verbs. This is a versatile activity that is easy to customize from the original paragraph and helps maintain the information learned.

Why Teach The Fill-In-The-Blanks Drill?

The "Fill-In-The-Blanks" drill is important for several reasons:

1. This is one way the therapist or parent can see how much the child is remembering. This is a particularly good exercise with children who find it very difficult to verbalize the correct answer in a structured sentence. If the child can write, then s/he can complete the drill on his/her own, thereby practicing independent work skills.
2. The information may be easier to remember when the child visualizes part of the answer.
3. The child begins to realize that decoding (reading without comprehending) is not going to work and that s/he must listen closely to the information in order to be successful at the drill.
4. In main stream settings at many different levels, children are required to complete "Fill In The Blank" exercises. Although these exercises may not be the best "yardstick" of comprehension, children are often required to complete these types of exercises; therefore, it is a good idea the teach the child the structure.

Samples of Animal Fill-In-The Blanks

The child should be presented with an animal "Fill-In" for every animal that s/he learns about. Each Fill-In-The-Blanks paragraph should be presented to the child in a large format and on separate sheets so that the child can easily read it; eventually, the child should learn to fill in the blanks by him/herself.

Fill in the blanks: Alligator   Date:_____

Alligators are _reptiles_. They grow to be 18 feet _long._. Alligators live in _swamps and rivers_. They have _big_ teeth and can be very _dangerous._. Alligators _swim_ very fast in the water. They _eat_ fish, snakes, and even small _mammals_ when they are hungry.

Fill in the blanks: Cats   Date:_____

There are many _different_ kinds of cats. Lions, jaguars, and _tigers_ are cats. The lion is called _king of the beasts_. It is a _meat_ eater. The jaguar is a _fast_ cat. It has yellow _fur_ and _brown_ spots. Jaguars _swim_ in the water and climb _trees_. Cheetahs are the _fastest_ runners. They live in the _trees_.

Fill in the blanks: Lizards   Date:_____

Lizards are _reptiles_. They are _cold_ blooded. There are many _different_ kinds of _lizards_. Most lizards are not big. They are _small_. Lizards have _four short_ legs. They are _fast_ runners. Lizards don't like to be cold; they like _warm_ weather. Lizards eat _insects and spiders_. Most _lizards_ lay eggs.

Fill in the blanks: Mammals   Date:_____

Mammals are _a group of animals_. They are _warm_ blooded. Mammals have a _backbone_. Some mammals eat _meat_ and some mammals eat _plants_. A _lion_ is a mammal. A _giraffe_ is a mammal.

Fill in the blanks: Reptiles   Date:_____

Reptiles are _a group of animals_. They are _warm_ blooded. Reptiles have a _backbone_. There are _many kinds_ of reptiles. Alligators, turtles, lizards, and _snakes_ are reptiles. Reptiles have _scaly_ skin. Most reptiles lay _eggs_. Some reptiles eat _meat_ and some eat _plants_. Some reptiles are tame, but some are _wild_.

Oral/Written Definitions

The Oral/Written Definition exercise is another activity designed to maintain information on animals. Once the child understands and assimilates the structured information about animals, the next stage is to give the child an opportunity to provide information about the animal of his/her choosing. The child should be able to provide a concise verbal definition of each animal s/he has learned. The definition should include the most important pieces of information about the animal, but may vary from week to week (e.g. a kangaroo is a marsupial that has a pouch; a kangaroo is an animal that lives in Australia). The child who has just been introduced to animal paragraphs will give very simple definitions such as "an elephant is an <u>animal</u> with a trunk". As the paragraphs become more difficult, the definitions should become more complex. An example of this is, "an elephant is a <u>mammal</u> with a trunk". Over time, the child should vary his/her definitions. If the child does not vary definitions without help, the therapist can model creativity by providing two definitions that are correct but different and then ask the child to do the same.

PROBLEMS: If the child has difficulty taking the information learned from the paragraph and placing it in the definitions, then the therapist should model the answer a few times with the child. At first, most of the definitions will be very similar. An example of this is, "an <u>(animal name)</u> is an animal with four legs". After the child learns the structure, s/he should be encouraged to include other, more distinctive characteristics about each animal. Examples include, "an elephant is an animal with a trunk" or "a giraffe is an animal with a long neck".

Why Teach Definitions?

Oral/written definitions are important because understanding the meaning of words is the key to children learning about their world. Normally developing children are constantly asking their parents to define things for them. Children with developmental disorders may be just as curious; however, they do not have a method by which they can easily find out about the world. Answering questions about definitions is a building block for asking questions about the world, and/or finding answers to questions through written material. Either way, the ability to use definitions is an important one. For the time being, these definitions are about animals; however, eventually a child with this skill may be able to apply it to other subjects.

Oral Definitions: Animals

The oral definition sheet should be introduced to the child once s/he has learned four animals. With every additional animal, the oral definition exercise can be used to learn about the new animal and maintain the information the child has acquired earlier about other animals. By combining animals that the child knows well with animals that s/he does not, the information is easily maintained. A few of the definitions are very easy and, therefore, highly motivating.

Oral Definitions: _Animals_

Give a definition of each animal by filling in the blanks.

Animals: _elephant_, _monkey_, _tiger_, _zebra_

1. A_n elephant_ is a_n animal_ with _a trunk_.

2. A _monkey_ is a_n animal_ with _a long tail_.

3. A _tiger_ is a_n animal_ that has _black and orange_
   stripes.

4. A _zebra_ is a_n animal_ that has _black and_
   white stripes.

Animal Grid Fill In

The therapist needs to work with the child to show him/her how to complete the animal grid. With practice, the child should begin to understand the structure of the grid and, hopefully, be able to complete it independently.

The therapist or parent should choose three animals to work with each time. The child should be able to generate the vital information on each animal because the information 1) has been presented before, and 2) is requested in a structured and specific form (in a grid). After all the information is written in the grid, the child should be required to verbally describe each animal in full sentences using the written information as a cue. Once the grid becomes relatively easy for the child, the animal comparison exercise introduced in the comparison section of this chapter should be introduced. If the grids are done on a weekly basis, the child will be able to more easily remember the information presented. The same format should be used for any new information that lends itself to this structure. Examples of other topics that can be introduced in this manner are given in the occupation and sport sections of this chapter.

Problems:
If the child is having difficulties with the grid, the therapist should prompt the child once, through an entire grid, using animals the child knows very well. If the child is still not picking up the structure, the therapist should use only one topic in the grid at first, using all three animals. Once the child understands the exercise using one category (such as "lives"), then the therapist should introduced the second category, until all four categories have been introduced.

When the child is able to do this grid independently, it can be adapted for many different kinds of general information.

 # Why Do This Drill?

As mentioned previously, children with developmental disorders tend to learn faster when there is a structure within which the information is presented. The grid is simply a way to give the child a template to organize the information that s/he must learn. The animal grid teaches children that the four main points about animals are their 1) category, 2) habitat, 3) nutrition, and 4) descriptive characteristic(s). Once the child has worked with the four main points for different species, s/he understands that they are important. When introduced to a group of animals in a noneducational setting, the child may learn through the natural environment because s/he will be interested in the topic and know what is important to observe. The goal is to teach the child to learn in much the same way as a typically developing peer would learn. Giving a portable structure to the child allows for greater educational independence.

Animal Grid Fill-In (Introduction to Animal Comparisons)

The Animal Grid Fill-In sheet should be introduced to the child once s/he has learned three animals. This exercise is somewhat harder than the definitions because the child must give four details about each animal; however, once the child understands the below structure, each animal will become progressively easier. This exercise can maintain the information the child has acquired previously by mixing newly introduced animals with familiar animals. Using this strategy should make the drill motivating because a few of the animals will be very easy to describe. Once the child becomes good at completing the grid, this exercise can be substituted with a more challenging comparison drill (see the section on comparisons in this chapter).

Animal Grid Fill-In

Fill in the blank boxes with what you know about each animal.

Animal	Duck	Snake	Lion
is	animal (bird - more advanced)	animal (reptile - more advanced)	animal (mammal - more advanced)
has	feathers	scales	a mane
lives	in or near water	all over the world	Africa
eats	plants and small animals	small animals	meat

How to Do the True or False Drill

Prerequisite: the child should be able to answer Yes/no questions about familiar items. Examples of Yes/No questions are, "Can you eat an apple?" or "Is a ball square?"

Once the child has a firm understanding of "Yes" and "No", the therapist can introduce true and false by pairing the words yes and no with true and false. This should be done using statements that the child knows to be either correct or incorrect. For example,
Therapist: "Is the sky blue?"
Child: "Yes."
Therapist: "Yes. That's TRUE."
(The therapist should then prompt the child to say, "Yes. That's True").
Child: "Yes. That's True."
The therapist should then make a statement from the same question.
Therapist: "The sky is blue."
(The therapist should then prompt the child to say, "True").
After several statements with the child being heavily prompted to say "True" or "False", the child will understand that True is related to "Yes", and that "False" is related to "No". If this is a problem, cue cards can be used and matched in such a way that the child puts True with Yes, and False with No.
Once the child can fairly accurately answer True/False to statements regarding topics that s/he is familiar with, then the therapist should have the child make false statements true. For example, "A ball is square" becomes "A ball is round" or "A block is square". The therapist should let the child physically correct the false statement by crossing out the incorrect word and writing a word that makes the statement true.

Initially, the therapist can let the child see the statement as she reads it. <u>Eventually, each statement should be presented verbally to the child, so that s/he must rely on his listening skills to be able to identify whether the statement is True or False.</u>

The therapist can and should use the True/False exercise with any new information recently presented to the child, including number comparisons, social scripts, concepts of time, definitions, and opposites such as hot/cold, wet/dry, and big/little. This exercise is one of many ways to check on the child's comprehension of any concept that has been already introduced.

A typical exercise would begin by the therapist slowly making the first statement. For example, "Ice-cream is hot." Then the therapist prompts, "False, because ice-cream is cold." If the child is not sure about the answer, the therapist should use her voice and face to prompt how ridiculous or untrue the statement is. The child may be uncertain about an answer because the statement is too difficult for the child. If that is the case, the therapist should choose easier statements. The therapist should go through the entire list of six statements in the same manner. It is important to make sure the child understands all the statements and the answers. ***This drill is NOT designed to teach the child facts; it is designed to teach the child the concept of true and false and test information the***

True or False Drill (Continued)

child has already learned through other exercises. The first few times the drill is done, the therapist may have to prompt the child. Once the child understands the concept of true and false, then the prompting should be eliminated. The first few drills should be done with obviously true or false statements. Once the child becomes good at this drill, then harder true or false questions should be added. It is important never to include "trick" questions. The point of the exercise is to teach the concept of true and false, not to frustrate the child.

The True or False drill is usually fun for the child; it is important that the therapist remember this when constructing the statements. During the first couple of months when the drill is introduced, the information the child has learned from the general information paragraphs (about animals, occupations, etc...) should be used. Once the therapist runs out of facts from these sources, general information statements the child knows can be used.

Why Teach True and False?

By introducing True and False into the comparison activity, the child is being taught to critically evaluate information being given to him/her. Because the information is familiar to the child, s/he is able to agree or disagree with the written statement. This is a foundation upon which to build critical thinking skills which are particularly important for children with developmental disorders.

True or False? (1)

The True or False exercise can include any information the child has **already learned**. The goal of this exercise is to hone the child's ability to differentiate between true and false because this ability to differentiate is a cornerstone to critical thinking. The True or False exercise is NOT designed to teach the child new information; rather, it is meant to be used with information that the child already has learned.

True or False?

Statement	If false, why...?
1. A giraffe is a fish.	False, because a giraffe is an mammal
2. A zebra has black and orange stripes.	False, because a zebra has black and white stripes.
3. A ladybug is an insect.	True.
4. Elephants live where it is cold	False, Elephants live where it is hot.
5. Lions eat plants and twigs.	False. Lions eat meat.
6. Chimpanzees live in Africa.	True.

True or False? (2)

This True or False exercise is a variation of the general true or false exercises. This exercise must include information the child knows well because the goal here is to strengthen the child's ability to discern between words that represent relative amounts such as most, much, or all. The goal of this exercise is to improve the child's ability to differentiate between these subtle true and false statements. This variation should only be done with the child once s/he understands the first True or False exercise very well.

True or False?

Use all, always, most, many, some, sometimes, few, never, etc. in the statement.

Statement	If false, why...?
1. Birds are always very colorful	False, because birds are sometimes very colorful.
2. All birds fly.	False, because most birds fly. A penguin does not fly.
3. Some birds eat paint.	False, because no birds eat paint.
4. Many birds have beaks.	False, because all birds have beaks.
5. Most birds lay eggs.	False, because all birds lay eggs.
A few birds do not fly.	True.

Topic Two: Occupations/Community Helpers

Prerequisite: The child should have already completed the section on animals.

The parent or therapist should read the paragraph slowly with feeling while sitting with the child at a table or on the floor (or wherever the child works). If the child can read, then s/he should follow along. Once the paragraph has been read, the therapist or child should read it again. If the child can read, it is a good opportunity to have him read it. Remember, the child should already be familiar with this structure from the animal paragraphs.

Then, the therapist should ask questions regarding the paragraph, and visually prompt the child, if necessary, by showing the child the place in the text where the answer lies. For example, if the first line reads, "An author is a person who writes something", the therapist should ask, "What does an author do?", and point to the first line. At first, the entire paragraph should be put into question form, in order. Once the child understands that the answer lies in the text, then s/he can be asked questions out of order. The idea is to teach the child that information can be obtained by reading; specifically, answers to factual questions can be found in text. This principle is important since it will teach the child comprehension, not just decoding. The child should have a fairly good understanding of this principle through his/her experience with the section on animals. The therapist can also have the child read the paragraph, and then ask questions about the paragraph without the child seeing the script. Once the child has mastered this skill (which may occur quickly or slowly, depending upon the age and reading ability of the child), then the therapist should read the script without showing the child what is written. In this way, the child must concentrate on understanding information being presented orally, a general weakness for most children with developmental disorders. Eventually, the child should be able to process the information in this way because the therapist has already given him/her the structure of what is being presented.

Information that is difficult will be better understood presented visually by having the child read the information; however, it is important to work on the child's auditory processing because much instruction and information is given verbally, particularly in mainstream educational settings.

Creating Occupation Scripts

When the professions have been depleted and the child shows an interest in a profession we have not included, the therapist or parent can create a new script by extracting four pieces of information that answer the following questions.

Who is a (<u>xxxxx</u>)? A (<u>xxxxx</u>) can be a man or a woman.

What does a (<u>xxxxx</u>) do?

Where does a (<u>xxxxx</u>) work? In an office, or a hospital or restaurant, etc.

What does a (<u>xxxxx</u>) wear or use? Some professions use a tool specific to their profession or wear a particular kind of uniform. Paragraphs on professions in which the members do not have a special uniform should not mention information on dress because this information does not differentiate the profession from other professions.

Occupations (Continued)

Occupation Drills: Do In Order

The following exercises are to be done in the following order. This order is designed to introduce the easier drills before the harder drills.
1. Outline For Topical Information
2. Fill-In-The-Blanks
3. Oral Definitions
4. Grid Fill-In
5. Who Would Say This?
6. What Would They Say?
7. True or False
8. Venn Diagram Comparisons
9. A Variety of Advanced Comparisons

Professions provided in this chapter include:
fire fighter, farmer, doctor, dentist, author, teacher, pilot, mailman, police officer.

Why Teach Occupations/Community Helpers?

This subject is very important because the child interacts often with these people in the community. This category can be very difficult for the child since occupations are somewhat abstract. It is a good idea to supplement the paragraph with pictures or actual experiences when possible. This category is important because typically developing children learn about occupations from an early age (particularly service occupations such as police officer, fire fighter, doctor, and dentist). Language delayed children may be lacking much general knowledge about professions because 1) we learn much about what someone does for a living auditorially 2) occupation is an abstract concept, and 3) the function of the occupation is not always readily apparent from the way the person dresses or behaves. This drill gives a clear structure about what constitutes the functions of common professions. A child needs to learn about occupations because 1) the child interacts with many members of "invasive" professions i.e. doctor, dentist, 2) information on occupations must be taught before learning about community since people in occupations make up the community, and 3) occupations are a common theme in elementary education.

How To Maintain Information on Professions

In order for the child to retain the information presented thus far, there are four activity work sheets that s/he should complete either verbally and/or in written form.

The four drills are:

1. Topical Outline
2. Fill in the Blanks
3. Oral Definitions
4. Verb Grid

Each of these drills is presented in this chapter with technique and explanation given.

Note: These paragraphs are much harder than the easiest paragraphs about animals. It is a good idea to wait until the child has mastered the animal paragraphs before introducing professions. If, however, there is an urgent need for the child to learn about different professions, then simplify the paragraphs by only including information about where the person works, what s/he does, what s/he uses, and what he wears.

Each paragraph below must be presented on a separate sheet in a larger format for easy reading and comprehension.

Samples

A Farmer

A farmer is a person who grows things. He lives and works on a farm.

Some farmers grow animals. They raise cows, chickens, pigs, and other animals. They milk the cows. They gather eggs from the chickens. They also feed the pigs and horses.

Some farmers grow plants. They grow things like vegetables, oats and wheat, and fruit.

Farmers use tractors and other machines to help them do their work.

Farmers are important to us. They grow food so that we can eat it.

Fire fighters

A fire fighter is a person who puts out fires. A fire fighter can be a man or a lady.

A fire fighter works at a fire station. When there is a fire someplace, fire fighters ride on fire trucks to the fire.

Fire fighters use special tools when they work. They use a hose and water to put out a fire. Sometimes they use an axe to get into a burning building.

A fire fighter wears special clothes. He wears a special hat, boots, pants, and a coat that protect him from the heat and flames of a fire.

Samples (Continued)

Chefs

A chef is a person who cooks food. A chef can be a man or a lady.

A chef works in a restaurant or hotel. He cooks all kinds of food, like meat, casseroles, vegetables, and desserts. A chef follows a recipe and prepares meals for people to eat.

Chefs use many different things when they work. They use silverware, pots and pans, and a stove or oven.

Chefs sometimes wear a white hat or an apron when they work.

Doctors

A doctor is a person who takes care of people who are sick or hurt. A doctor can be a man or a lady.

There are many different kinds of doctors. There are eye doctors, heart doctors, and bone doctors.

Doctors work in a hospital or in an office.

Doctors use many special tools when they work. A doctor uses a stethoscope to listen to your heart. A doctor uses a thermometer to take your temperature. Sometimes, a doctor will give you medicine if you are sick.

Doctors are very important. If you are sick or hurt, a doctor will help you get better.

Dentists

A dentist is a person who takes care of your teeth. A dentist can be a man or a lady.

A dentist works in an office.

A dentist uses many special tools when he works. He uses a mirror to look in your mouth. He has a special chair that you sit in. If your tooth has a cavity or hole in it, the dentist will fix it.

A dentist will tell you to brush your teeth after you eat. He will tell you not to eat candy or other sweets because they are not good for your teeth.

How To Introduce Topical Outlines

Prerequisite: The child should already be familiar with all the exercises used to introduce animals. Even if the child is quite old, we strongly recommend that the general information section on animals be taught since that is the most concrete subject used in this book and therefore, the easiest way to introduce the child to the various structures we provide. The topical outlines should be introduced in the same way as they were when animals were introduced.

First, the therapist should have the child read the paragraph she has chosen for the child. Next, the therapist should read the paragraph to the child. The therapist should have the outline already completed using only one word to represent a point about the occupation. Then, the therapist should have the child read about the paragraph from the outline. The child should use an entire sentence based on each key word. Initially, the child will need to be prompted. The therapist can point to the name of the profession to prompt the child, or she can model the short sentence using emphasis e.g. A DOCTOR works in an OFFICE. Once the child can make full sentences from the outline, the child should be asked to tell the therapist about the occupation without the outline.

When the child becomes good at this exercise, s/he can help the therapist fill in the outline using key words. For an example of the verbal interchange between therapist and child, please refer to the first "How To Teach Topical Outlines" section for animals.

Once the child has done the topical outline with the therapist several times on a particular paragraph, it is time to introduce the Simple Child-Generated Outline. This next drill (the Simple Outline) has the child tell the therapist about the paragraph without the therapist completing a topical outline. The therapist asks the child, "What is the paragraph about?", and writes down the child's answer under Topic. Then the therapist says, "Tell me about (topic)". The therapist prompts the child to tell her three things and writes them under "details". Then, the child uses this outline to speak about the topic in complete sentences.

Once the child can do this easily, the "Simple Outline With Elaborative Statement" drill can be introduced. The therapist goes through the sheet as with the Simple Outline, but this time she says, "Tell me something about (the detail)". This constitutes the elaborative statement. The child then uses his/her outline to talk about the topic.

Once the child is comfortable with elaborative statements, the therapist should introduce the Multi-Paragraph Outline. It is important to make sure that 1) the child has fully grasped elaborative statements and is ready for this advanced exercise and 2) the child knows enough about the topic to write a multi-paragraph outline (based on all the paragraphs read prior to this level). The therapist begins the exercise by asking the child to identify the topic and some details about the topic. Then she asks the child to give examples of the topic. Each example becomes the topic of a paragraph. Then, the child must provide three details about each example. Finally, the child uses his multi-paragraph outline to communicate about the topic. *Note: With a verbal child always do the verbal drill with and without the outline.*

Why Teach Topical Outlines

Topical outlines make the structure of the paragraph explicit. Eventually, the child may take other paragraphs and organize them in a way that is easy to understand and memorize. In addition, the topical outline can be used as a crutch for those children who have difficulty in verbalizing a complete sentence. The right type of word (e.g. verb or noun) acts to prompt the rest of the sentence. Even though this drill is highly structured and patterned, it promotes talking.

Outline For Topical Information

This exercise teaches the child how to comprehend text and differentiate between main idea and detail. The outline should be completed by the therapist before the session begins. First, the child reads the paragraph. Then, the therapist uses the outline to help the child comprehend and talk about the paragraph. Eventually the child should be able to tell the therapist what information should be included in the outline.

Outline For Topical Information

Topic: _Farmer_

Main Idea: _A farmer grows things_

Details: _works   farm_

plants

vegetables

cows

horses

pigs

eggs

tractor

Simple Child - Generated Outline

This exercise teaches the child how to organize information. The outline should be completed by the child during the session. First, the child reads the paragraph. Then, s/he dictates the information to the therapist. Initially, the child should only be expected to give one word. Eventually, the child should be able to tell the therapist about the topic in complete sentences by using these words as prompts. Once the child has mastered this exercise, s/he should be given the opportunity to write a short paragraph based on his/her outline.

Simple Outline For Topical Information

Topic: _____farmers_____

Tell me about _____farmers_____

Main Idea: _____grows things_____

Details: _____works farm_____

_____tractor_____

_____cows_____

Simple Outline with Elaborative Statement

This exercise teaches the child how to comprehend and organize information. This outline, like the simple outline, should be completed by the child during the session. First, the child reads the paragraph. Then, the child should dictate the information to the therapist. The child should give a detail from the paragraph and then elaborate on that detail. Once the child has mastered the outline with elaborative statement, s/he should be given the opportunity to write a short paragraph based on his/her outline.

Outline For Topical Information (Elaborative)

Topic: __farmers__

Tell me about __farmers__

Main Idea: __grows things__

__corn, peas, beans__

__works farm__

__gets dirt ready__

__tractor__

__hay__

__cows__

__milk__

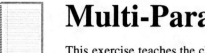

Multi-Paragraph Outline

This exercise teaches the child how to comprehend and organize information from a written text. The outline should be completed by the child during the session. First, the child reads the paragraph. Then, the child dictates the information to the therapist. The child should tell the therapist the topic of the paragraph, and give a few details about the topic. Then, the child should be prompted to give examples of the topic. Those examples become the main idea for the smaller paragraphs. Next, the child should be asked to come up with three details for each secondary topic. Finally, the child should be able to talk about the topic using this outline.

Multi-Paragraph Outline For Topical Information

Topic: _____ Farmer _____

General Info: _____ works farm _____

_____ countryside _____

_____ grows things _____

1. Topic: _____ lives _____

Details: _____ house _____

_____ barn _____

_____

3. Topic: _____ animals _____

Details: _____ cows _____

_____ chickens _____

_____ horses _____

2. Topic: _____ tractor _____

Details: _____ drives _____

_____ dirt _____

_____ hay _____

4. Topic: _____ plants _____

Details: _____ corn _____

_____ wheat _____

_____

How To Use Profession Fill-In-The-Blanks

After the therapist and child have read a paragraph and completed a topical outline, the "Fill-In-The-Blank" exercise can be introduced. The therapist should read the sentences to the child and stop before every space. The child should be prompted to fill in the blank. The blanks can be customized to target the child's weaknesses. To illustrate, a child with difficulty using verbs can be required to complete a "Fill in the Blanks" drill where all the spaces are verbs. This is a versatile activity that is easy to customize from the original paragraph to incorporate any general knowledge.

Why Introduce This Drill?

As we explained in the section on Animal Fill-In-The-Blanks, this exercise gives the therapist another way to focus the child's attention towards what is important in the paragraph. The "Fill-In-The-Blank" drill is important for several reasons:
1. This is one way the therapist or parent can see how much the child remembers from a paragraph. It is particularly good for children who find it very difficult to verbalize the correct answer. In addition, if the child can write, then s/he can complete the drill on his/her own which is good for independent work skills.
2. The information may be easier to remember when the child visualizes part of the answer.
3. The child begins to realize that decoding (reading without comprehending) is not effective and that s/he really must listen to the information in order to be successful at the drill.
4. In a main stream setting, children are often required to complete fill in the blank exercises.

Samples of Occupation Fill-In-The-Blanks

The child should be presented with an occupation Fill In The Blank exercise for every profession that s/ he learns about. Each Fill In The Blanks paragraph should be presented to the child in large format so that the child can easily read it and eventually learn to fill in the blanks him/herself.

Fill in the blanks: Doctor
Date:_____

A doctor is a ___person___ who takes care of people who are ___sick___ or ___hurt___. A doctor can be a ___a man___ or a lady. There are many different kinds of ___doctors___. There are ___eye___ doctors, ___heart___ doctors, or bone doctors. Doctors work in an office or ___hospital___. Doctors use many special ___tools___ when they work. A doctor uses a ___stethoscope___ to listen to your heart. A doctor uses a ___thermometer___ to take your temperature. Sometimes, a doctor will give you ___medicine___ if you are sick.

Doctors are very important. If you are sick or ___hurt___, a ___doctor___ will help you get better.

Fill in the blanks: Dentist
Date:_____

A dentist is a ___person___ who takes care of your ___teeth___. A dentist can be a man or a ___lady___. A dentist uses many special ___tools___ when he works. He uses a ___mirror___ to look in your mouth. If your tooth has a ___cavity___ or hole in it, the dentist will fix it. A dentist will tell you to ___brush your teeth___ after you eat. He will tell you not to eat ___candy___ or other sweets because they are not good for your teeth.

Fill in the blanks: Fire fighter
Date:_____

A fire fighter is a ___person___ who puts out ___fires___. A fire fighter can be ___a man___ or ___a lady___.

A ___fireman___ works at a fire ___station___. When there is a fire someplace, fire fighters ride on ___a fire truck___ to the fire.

Fire fighters use ___special tools___ when they work. They use a ___hose___, and ___water___ to put out a fire. Fire fighters wear a special ___hat___, ___boots___, ___pants___, and ___coat___ to protect them from the heat and flames of the ___fire___.

Fill in the blanks: Carpenter
Date:_____

A carpenter is a ___person___ who builds ___houses___ and other things made of wood. Carpenters are usually ___men___. Some carpenters build ___houses___, some build ___furniture___, and some ___build___ decks. A carpenter works ___outside___ at a work site, or in a ___woodshop___. Carpenters use many different ___tools___. They use a ___saw___, ___a hammer___, a measuring tape, and a screwdriver. A carpenter wears old ___clothes___ and gets ___very dirty___.

Fill in the blanks: Chefs
Date:_____

A chef is a ___person___ who cooks ___food___. A chef can be a man or ___a lady___. A chef works in ___a restaurant___ or hotel. He cooks all kinds of food, like ___meat___, casseroles, ___vegetables___, and desserts. A chef follows a recipe and prepares ___meals___ for people to eat.

Chefs use ___pots___, ___silverware___, and ___an oven or stove___ when they work.

Chefs sometimes wear a ___hat or apron___ when they work.

Oral/Written Definitions

This is the next stage of maintaining information learned about professions. Once the child understands and assimilates the structured information about professions, this step gives him/her an opportunity to use the professions of the his/her choosing. The child should be able to provide a concise verbal definition of each profession s/he has learned. The definition should include the most important pieces of information about the profession, but may vary from week to week (e.g. a dentist is a person that checks your teeth; a dentist is a person who uses special tools). Over time, the child should be encouraged to vary the definitions. If the child does not vary definitions without help, the therapist can provide 2 definitions that are correct but different and then ask the child to do the same.

Problems: If the child has difficulty taking the information learned from the grid and placing it in the definitions, then the therapist should model the answer a few times for the child. At first, most of the definitions will be very similar i.e. a (xxxxx) is an person who (xxxxx). After the child learns the structure, s/he should be encouraged to include other more distinctive characteristics about each profession i.e. a doctor uses a stethoscope, a carpenter uses a saw, a measuring tape and a screwdriver.

 # Why Teach Definitions?

Oral/written definitions are important because children with developmental delays need concepts made explicit for them to learn auditory information about their world. Normally developing children are constantly asking their parents to define things for them. Developmentally delayed children may be just as curious; however, they do not have an outlet or method by which they can easily find out about the world. Ability to answer questions about definitions may be a prerequisite to asking questions about the world, or being self-sufficient to find answers about questions through written material. Either way, the ability to use definitions is an important one. The definitions which the children give are very structured for the time being; however, eventually a child with this skill may use the ability to define other topics and make better sense of the world.

Oral Definitions: Occupations

The oral definition sheet can be introduced to the child once s/he has studied four occupations. With every additional occupation introduced, the oral definition exercise can be used to solidify the new occupation and maintain the information the child has already acquired. By adding occupations that the child knows well, with occupations that s/he does not, the information is easily remembered and the more familiar definitions become very easy and highly motivating.

Oral Definitions: _Occupations_

Give a definition of each occupation by filling in the blanks.

Occupation: _carpenter_ , _dentist_ , _doctor_ , _farmer_

1. A _carpenter_ is a _person_ who _builds houses_ .

2. A _dentist_ is a _person_ who _takes care of your teeth_ .

3. A _doctor_ is a _person_ who _helps when you are sick or hurt_ .

4. A _farmer_ is a _person_ who _grows things._ .

Occupation Grid Fill-In

The therapist should introduce this exercise by showing the child how to fill in the occupation grid. The child will quickly begin to understand the structure of the grid and then be able to complete the grid by him/herself.

The therapist or parent should choose three professions to use each time. The child should be able to generate the vital information on each occupation because 1) the information has been presented before and 2) the information grid is structured and specific. After all information is written on the grid, the child should verbally describe each profession using the information as a cue to help form complete sentences. Once the verbal description becomes relatively easy for the child, the child should be introduced to occupation comparisons. If these are done on a weekly basis, the child will be better able to retain the information studied. The same format should be used for all new information that lends itself to this structure.

Problems

If the child has difficulties with the grid, the therapist should prompt the child through an entire grid several times, using professions the child knows very well. Remember, the child should be very familiar with the format because it is almost identical to the format used for animals. If the child still does not understand the structure, the therapist should use only one topic in the grid at first, but use all three professions. Once the child understands the structure with one category i.e. uses, then the therapist should introduced the second category until all four categories have been introduced.

 # Why Do This Drill?

As we have mentioned previously, children with pervasive developmental disorders tend to learn faster when there is a structure within which the information is presented. The grid is simply a way to give these children a template to organize the information that they must learn. The professions grid teaches children five important points about professions: their category (who they are); what they do; where they work; what they use; and descriptive characteristics such as what they wear or look like. Once the child grasps the concept of professions, s/he will be more likely to be aware of professions in a noneducational setting. The child has a better chance of learning through his/her natural environment because s/he already knows something about the topic. The goal is to prepare the child to learn in much the same way as a non-developmentally delayed peer would learn. Giving a portable structure to the child enables educational independence.

Occupation Grid Fill-In (Introduction to Occupation Comparisons)

The Occupation Grid Fill-In sheet should be introduced to the child once s/he has learned three occupations. The child has already been introduced to the structure when learning about animals. The addition of occupations the child knows well (to ones that s/he is just learning), easily maintains the familiar information and highly motivates the child since the child finds part of the exercise easy. Once the child is good at this easy comparison, more difficult comparisons can be substituted (see the end of this chapter).

Occupation Grid Fill-In

Fill in the blank boxes with what you know about each occupation.

Job	Doctor	Chef	Farmer
is a person who	helps people who are sick or hurt	cooks food	grows food, and raises animals
works	in a hospital or office	in a restaurant or hotel	on a farm
uses	a stetho-scope	a stove and an oven	a tractor
wears/ does	gives medicine	a white apron	gets eggs from the chickens

"Who Would Say This?" and "What Would They Say?" Drill

Once the child has learned about several occupations, the next step is to incorporate this knowledge into a practical form. The "Who Would Say This?" drill attempts to do this. The therapist should have the child identify the profession that a particular phrase is associated with. For example, the dentist says, "Don't eat candy" or "Brush your teeth", or the fire fighter says, "Don't play with matches". The completed drill is provided to give the parent or therapist an idea of what kind of statements the person would make in the occupations introduced. The statements should be obvious at first, so the child understands the drill. As the child gets older, these statements can be augmented; however, in the beginning, it is wise to stick to the cliche statements. *Note: The phrases that the professional says should relate to social rules when possible.*

The "What Would They Say" drill has the child think about the role of the profession and come up with a typical statement for that profession. Stereotypical answers are acceptable in this exercise. This exercise becomes very difficult and loses its purpose if the child must actually come up with original statements.

These drills can also be used in pretend play. The child and peer can act out the role of dentist and patient, for example, to make the phrases the professional says more relevant.

Why Teach This Drill?

The point of these drills is twofold: first, the child needs to understand how these professions relate to him/her. For example, the role of a dentist is defined through various statements a dentist would make. If the child expects the dentist to talk about teeth brushing or flossing, the child comes to understand the role of the dentist through 1) the general information paragraphs, 2) the Who Would Say This drill, and 3) the What Would They Say drill. After the child learns about dentists from these activities, hopefully the trip to the dentist becomes less mysterious. The second goal of this drill is to maintain general knowledge about the dentist, learned from the paragraph introduced earlier.

Who Would Say This?

This exercise has the child identify the occupation based on what a member of that occupation would say. This drill should be introduced only when the child has learned about eight occupations from the paragraphs. Some occupations are harder to identify than others. The easy questions must be included to give the child the opportunity to successfully answer some of the questions unprompted. If the child has difficulty giving an answer, it is important to prompt the child to guarantee success.

Who Would Say This?

Read the directions:

You have learned about a ___*dentist*___, ___*fire fighter*___, ___*teacher*___, ___*waiter/ess*___ ___*doctor*___, ___*carpenter*___, ___*author*___, ___*mailman*___ .

You should know what each person might say.

Read what is said and write down WHO would say it on the line. The first one is done for you.

Who?		Says What?
1.	*"Dentist"*	"Don't eat candy."
2.	*Fire fighter*	"Don't play with matches."
3.	*Teacher*	"Do your homework."
4.	*Server*	"May I take your order?"
5.	*Dentist*	"Brush your teeth".
6.	*Doctor*	"Let me take your temperature."
7.	*Doctor*	"Where does it hurt?"
8.	*Carpenter*	"Pass me the hammer."

What Would They Say?

This exercise is designed to take the knowledge the child has gained from the occupation paragraphs and make him/her critically think about what members of each occupation say. This is a difficult exercise because the child has to think about what members of the occupation do, and then think of something that those members would say that is relevant to the occupation.

What Would They Say?

Read the directions:

You have learned about a ___doctor___ , ___dentist___ , ___fire fighter___ , ___waiter/ess___, ___clerk___ , ___carpenter___, ___chef___ , ___policeman___ .

You should know who says what.

Read the name of the job and write down what each occupation would say on the line. The first one is done for you.

Who?	Says What?
1. Doctor	"Where does it hurt?"
2. Dentist	Don't eat candy
3. Fire fighter	don't play with matches
4. Waiter	May I take your order
5. Clerk	How can I help you
6. Carpenter	pass me the hammer
7. Chef	don't burn the food
8. Policeman	don't talk to strangers

Topic Three: Places In The Community

The first step to teaching about places in the community is to read about a community with the child so s/he knows what a community is. There are two versions of the community script -- Easy and Difficult. The child should be introduced to the Easy script first. Once the child's reading comprehension skills increase, the Difficult script can be introduced. Teaching about various places in the community should be done in the same way as the animals and professions topics were taught using oral definitions, topical outlines, and grids. For places in the community, the important information is what happens in the place (e.g. what is its purpose), who works in the place, what one would go to the place to do (e.g. watch a sporting event), and characteristics of the place (e.g. a stadium is loud, big, and round).

Drills To Do In Order

1. Introduction of Community Script
2. Outline For Topical Information for script
3. Introduction of the Places in the Community paragraphs
4. Fill-In-The-Blanks
5. Oral Definitions
6. Grid Fill-In
7. True or False
8. Venn Diagram Comparisons
9. A Variety of Advanced Comparisons

The "Introduction of Community" Script and samples of "Places in the Community" follow. The drills 2 through 7 listed above have been explained at the beginning of the chapter in the "Animals" and "Occupations" units. Drills 8 and 9 are described in detail in the "Comparisons" section near the end of the chapter.

Why Teach About Community?

This topic is very important for the child to learn for several reasons. Community information is general knowledge that normally developing children pick up auditorially at a young age. In addition, knowledge about the community is a prerequisite for creating an independent adult who can live comfortably in the community. Also, the community is a large part of most children's lives. Since the community is all around us, it is a good topic to discuss and build upon.

Community Scripts

Once the child has learned about animals and occupations (which probably has taken the better part of a year if not longer, depending on the child's age and ability), then it is time to introduce community. The Easy Community Script should be introduced first, using the same technique as was used to introduce the animal and occupation paragraphs. All of the various drills that were used with animals and occupations should be adapted to community. Once the child has learned about a community, then the places in the community should be introduced.

My Community (Easy)

A community is the group of people and all the things in an area or place. There are many kinds and sizes of communities.

My community is made up of all the people, places and things in my neighborhood and city.

My community has lots of different people. Doctors, dentists, the mailman, the garbage man, the clerks at the store, and the people that work at McDonald's and Burger King are in my community.

There are many different places in my community. There are buildings, lakes, parks and stores in my community. Safeway, Longs, and Mervyn's are stores in my community.

There are many different things in my community. There are streets and roads, cars, trucks and bridges. There are also many different plants and animals. I see things in my community everywhere I look.

My Community (Difficult)

A community is the group of people and all the things in a certain area or place. There are many kinds and sizes of communities. The most important community for me to know about is my own community.

My community is made up of all the people, places and things in my neighborhood and the city of (where ever the child lives) .

My community has lots of different people. The people in my family and my neighbors all live in my community. Community helpers and workers like doctors, dentists, the mailman, the garbage man, the clerks at the store, and the people that work at McDonald's and Burger King are all part of my community.

There are many different places in my community. There are buildings, lakes, and parks. Safeway, Longs, and Mervyn's are stores in my community. Tanforan Mall is part of my community, too. The bank, many restaurants, gas stations, and movie theaters are all part of the area where I live. Crystal Lake, the YMCA, and the public library are three more places in my community.

There are many different things in my community. There are streets and roads, signs and lights, cars, trucks, buses and bridges. There are also many different plants and animals. I see things that are part of my community everywhere that I look.

Samples of Places in the Community

A Post Office

A post office is a place where you mail a letter or package. A mailman works in a post office. He picks up letters and packages at the post office. Then, he brings them to people's houses and puts them in their mailboxes.

A post office has machines that sell you stamps. You can also buy a stamp from a mailman at the post office. The post office has scales to weigh your letter or package.

When you are ready to mail a letter, you put a stamp on it and put the letter in a slot at the post office for the mailman to pick up. When you mail a package, you give it to the mailman at the counter at the post office. It costs money to mail a package.

You can mail a letter or package to anyone anywhere in the world. Just bring it to the post office, and the letter or package will be sent to the person you want it to go to.

A Stadium

A stadium is a place where you can watch sports. It has a big field with many rows of seats around it.

Many people can fit in a stadium. A stadium is very big.

You can watch baseball or football or soccer in a stadium. You can also buy things to eat there.

A stadium can be very noisy. When a baseball or football game is being played in a stadium, people cheer loudly.

A Bank

A bank is a place where people keep their money. Bank of America, Royal Bank, and Bank of the West are names of banks.

Many people work in a bank. The person who takes your money and puts it somewhere safe is called a bank teller.

You can put money in the bank, or you can take your money out of the bank when you need to.

When you go to a bank, you usually have to wait in line to see a bank teller. When it is your turn, you give the teller some money and a piece of paper that tells how much money you are putting in the bank. Or, you give the teller a piece of paper that tells how much money you are taking out of the bank.

If you want to save money and make sure that it is safe, put it in a bank.

Topic Four: Sports

Sports is an important topic for children who are mainstreamed and must participate in physical education. If the child learns about the rules of a sport before s/he has to participate, then it will be much easier for the child to learn the sport when it is introduced to the group. The basic vocabulary and goal of each sport is introduced in the scripts. By introducing the child to the sport in this way, the child knows what s/he is supposed to do beforehand.   For the child who is coordinated, organized sports can be a good way to integrate him/her into a group of typically developing children. Sport scripts should contain the basic characteristics of the sport such as where it is played, what you need to play the sport (e.g. a bat, a ball or a racket), the basic rules, the goal of the game, and how one wins the game.

Sports Drills To Do In Order

The exercises are done in the same way as with the preceding topics. They should be done in the following order:
1. Outline For Topical Information
2. Fill-In-The-Blanks
3. Oral Definitions
4. Grid Fill-In
5. True or False
6. A Variety of Advanced Comparisons
7. Which Sport Goes With Which Description?

Samples of "Sports" paragraphs follow. The drills 1 through 5 listed above have been explained at the beginning of the chapter in the "Animals" and "Occupations" units. Drills 6 and 7 are described in detail in the "Comparisons" section near the end of the chapter.

Why Teach About Sports?

This topic is a good one for the child to learn since throughout school in gym class, the child will be required to take part in these sports. The reality is, however, that Sport scripts are much more important for boys than girls since a boy who cannot play sports is stigmatized to a greater extent than a girl who cannot play sports. An active girl can benefit from these scripts as well if the relevant ones are chosen (baseball rather than football). Sports teams are a good way for the child to form a peer group if the child is at all physically capable and interested in the game.

Samples of Sport Paragraphs

Basketball

Basketball is a team sport. It is a game.

You play basketball with a big, round ball. You play basketball on a basketball court.

A basketball game is played between two teams. There are five players on each basketball team.

When you play basketball, you dribble or bounce the ball down the basketball court. You can pass or throw the ball to someone on your team.

In basketball, you try to throw the ball through a basketball hoop. The hoop is up high. The hoop is round and has a net.

When you make a basket, you score two points. In basketball, the team with the most points at the end of the game wins.

Baseball

Baseball is a team sport. It is a game.

You play baseball on a baseball field. The baseball field has lots of grass. The infield has grass and dirt, and it has a 1st base, 2nd base, 3rd base, and home plate.

You need a ball, a bat, and a glove to play baseball. Sometimes, you wear a helmet or hat and a uniform.

A baseball game is played between two teams. There are nine players on each baseball team.

One team hits or bats the ball, and the other team catches or fields the ball. The team hitting the ball tries to get to 1st base, then 2nd base, then 3rd base, then home plate. The team catching or fielding the ball tries to get the team at bat out. When there are 3 outs, the teams change places.

Every time the team at bat runs around the bases and gets to home plate, it scores 1 run. The team with the most runs at the end of the game wins.

Samples of Sport Paragraphs (Continued)

Soccer

Soccer is a team sport. It is a game.

You can play soccer indoors or outdoors. You play soccer on a soccer field. The field is large, and it is in the shape of a rectangle.

You need a soccer ball to play soccer. Sometimes you wear a uniform and special shoes.

A soccer game is played between two teams. There are 11 players on each team. There are 3 forwards, 3 mid-fielders, 4 defenders, and 1 goalie.

In soccer, you can kick the ball or strike the ball with your head or body. You try to kick the ball to the other players on your team. You can not pick up the ball with your hands. Only the goalie can touch the ball with his hands. In soccer, you cannot kick or push another player.

In soccer, you try to score a goal. You try to kick or strike the soccer ball into the other team's goal area. The goal area usually has a net. The goalie on the other team tries to block the ball from entering the goal area. If you kick or strike the ball into the net, you score a goal. A goal is worth 1 point. The team that scores the most goals at the end of the game wins.

Football

Football is a team sport. It is a game.

You play football on a football field. The field is large and long. At each end of the football is an end zone. There is a goal post in each end zone.

You need a football, helmet, pads, and a uniform to play football. You need a helmet and pads because football is a rough sport. You can get hurt if you are not careful.

A football game is played between two teams. There are lots of players on each football team. But, only 11 players from each team can play on the field at a time.

A football team has 2 units or groups of players. One group is called the Offensive Unit. The Offensive Unit tries to score. The quarterback is on the Offensive Unit. He is the leader. The other group of players is called the Defensive Unit. The Defensive Unit tries to stop the other team from scoring. Players on the Defensive Unit try to tackle the person with the ball.

In football, you can pass the ball, run with the ball, or kick the ball.

In football, teams try to score points. Each team tries to carry the ball across the goal line and into the end zone. A team can score a touchdown, an extra point, or a field goal. A touchdown is worth 6 points. An extra point is worth 1 point. A field goal is worth 3 points. The team with the most points at the end of the football game wins.

Samples of Sports Fill-in-The-Blanks

The child should be presented with a Sports Fill-In for every sport that s/he learns about. Each Fill-In-The-Blanks paragraph should be presented to the child in a large format so that the child can easily read it and eventually learn to fill in the blanks him/herself. The Sports Fill-In exercise should be introduced to the child in the same way as the animal and occupation Fill-In-The-Blanks exercises.

Fill in the blanks: Basketball
Date:_____

Basketball is a ___team___ sport. It is a _game_.
You play basketball with a __big, round, orange ball__. You play basketball on a __basketball court__.

A basketball game is played between __two teams__. There are __5__ players on each team.   You ___dribble___ or ___bounce___ a basketball.

In basketball, you try to throw the ball through a ___basketball hoop___. The hoop has a net.

A basket scores ___2___ points. The team with the most ___points___ at the end of the game wins.

Fill in the blanks: Baseball
Date:_____

Baseball is a ___team___ sport. It is a _game_.
You play baseball on a ___baseball field___. The field has an ___infield___ and an ___outfield___.

You need a ___ball___, ___bat___, and ___glove___ to play baseball.

A baseball game is played between ___two teams___. There are ___9___ players on each team. One team hits or ___bats___ the ball, and the other team catches or ___fields___ the ball.

When the team at bat runs around 1st, 2nd, and 3rd base and gets to home plate, it scores _1_ run. The team with the most ___runs___ wins the game.

Fill in the blanks: Soccer
Date:_____

Soccer is a ___team___ sport. It is a _game_.
You play soccer __indoors or outdoors__. You play _soccer_ on a soccer field. The field is __large__ and in the shape of a __rectangle__.

You need a _soccer ball_ to play soccer. Sometimes you wear a _uniform_ and special _shoes_.

A soccer game is played between _two teams_. There are _11_ players on each team. There are _3_ forwards, _3_ midfielders, _3_ defenders, and 1 _goalie_.

In Soccer, you can _kick_ the ball or strike the ball with your head or body. You cannot _pick up_ the ball with your hands. Only the _goalie_ can touch the ball with his hands. In _soccer_, you cannot kick or push another _player_.

In _soccer_, you try to score a _goal_. You try to kick or strike the _ball_ into the other _term's_ goal area. The goal area usually has a net. The goalie on the other _team_ tries to block the ball from entering the _goal area_. If you kick or strike the ball into the net, you score a _goal_.
A goal is worth _1_ point. The team that scores the most _goals_ at the end of the game _wins_.

Other Topics

Other topics, such as those featured below, should be introduced and maintained in the same way as the topics previously introduced in this chapter.

Topic Five: Planets

Teaching about planets should be done in the same way as animals and professions were taught, using: (1) oral definitions, (2) topical outlines, (3) grids, and (4) comparisons. For planets, the important information is: size, color, order from sun, gas or rock, and distinctive features such as rings, and number of moons.

Topic Six: Geography

Teaching about geography should be done in the same way as animals and professions were taught, using: (1) oral definitions, (2) topical outlines, (3) grids, and (4) comparisons. For geography, the important information is: continents, countries, capitals; and mountains, oceans, life, relative location, weather, distinctive features.

Topic Seven: Habitats

Teaching about various habitats should be done in the same way as animals and professions, using: (1) oral definitions, (2) topical outlines, (3) grids, and (4) comparisons. For habitats, the salient information is: what/who lives there, descriptions (location, features).

Why Teach These Topics?

There are a virtually infinite number of topics that can be used to teach general knowledge. The above topics are common ones that the child is going to come across if s/he is mainstreamed. It is a good idea to prepare the child for these topics so that when they are taught in school, s/he will be more inclined to listen to group instruction on the topic because it is familiar. Other topics should be introduced to the child if 1) there is interest on the part of the child, and 2) the knowledge is going to be directly applicable to the child's life i.e. the child is going to join a team, club, or class which engages in ,or learns about, a particular activity.

How To Create Information Paragraphs

There are a few steps to go through in order to create information paragraphs for teaching general knowledge. Once the parent or therapist acquires this skill, any topic that the child needs to learn about can be introduced in this way.

1. From a children's dictionary, the following should be extracted: A (name of topic) is a (general category) that (uses or does). This should be 1 or 2 sentences.

Some examples: A lion is a mammal that lives in Africa.
A doctor is a person who helps people feel better.
A store is a place where we buy things.
A country is a place where people live (map required).
A desert is land that is very dry.
The solar system is a place with 9 planets (picture required).

2. The next 1 to 3 sentences should describe the features of the topic. The sentences should be about the most obvious, generally accepted features of the topic. Refer to the paragraphs in this chapter for examples of the items to be included.

3. Following the descriptive sentence(s), there should be 1 or 2 sentences which answer a "where" question i.e. "Where does the animal live?", or "Where does the doctor work?". The "where" information should be both general and detailed, particularly as the paragraphs become more difficult e.g. a chimpanzee lives in Africa (general) but it also lives in a zoo or in the jungle (detailed).

4. Finally, the paragraph should include a sentence which describes another aspect of the topic such as what the animal eats, or what the professional does.

Each thought should be in a different paragraph even if the entire description is only 6 sentences long. It is important to indent each new paragraph to show that the sentence begins a new paragraph. All our descriptive paragraphs are indented in this way (aside from the very easiest animal paragraphs). By giving each new thought a paragraph of its own, the child learns that each paragraph has only one main idea. There are many books that have paragraphs already completed; however, in order to use paragraphs from published books, they must be simplified. The long term goal is for the child to graduate from customized paragraphs to published books; however, this goal will take years to achieve. Prematurely introducing the child to a level s/he cannot handle will frustrate him/her and set up the situation for possible failure; therefore, it is CRITICAL to use customized paragraphs for as long as necessary.

Why Customize Paragraphs?

Once the child can learn information through paragraphs, s/he can be introduced to any topic s/he needs to know. The ability to create information paragraphs gives the parent or therapist a powerful teaching tool. Some children can eventually use easy paragraphs found in books to learn about a subject; however, some children will need to have customized paragraphs presented to them in perpetuity. Therefore, it is important that those who work with the child have the ability to customize paragraphs.

Current Topics

This record sheet is designed to give the therapist a sense of how quickly or slowly the child is progressing through the paragraphs, and which paragraphs have been covered and need to be reviewed.

Current Topics

Date	Theme	Topic	Info. Child Should Know (for all topics)
9/95	Animals	Bears	What they are.
		Monkeys	Where they live.
		Giraffes	What they eat.
		Lions	What they have.
		Ducks	
1/96	Occupations	Doctor	What they do.
		Dentist	Where they work.
		Carpenter	What they use.
		Fire fighter	What they wear.
		Chef	Why they are important.
6/96	Community	Community	General
		Post Office	What it has
		Bank	Who works there
		Stadium	How one uses it
		Library	What is the purpose
9/96	Sports	Soccer	What it is
		Basketball	Where it is played
		Football	What you need to play
		Baseball	What the basic rules are
		Hockey	How you win

Comparisons (Easy)

Venn Diagram Comparisons

Venn Diagrams are the first type of comparison to be introduced because these diagrams are good visual representations of comparisons. We suggest the reader view the example given on the following page while reading the "How To" portion below.

The first time the child does this exercise, the sheet should be completed and the child should be prompted to do the exercise. The therapist can model the exercise for the child if s/he has difficulty in understanding what to do. The exercise is done in the following manner:

The therapist must choose two animals to compare (or two objects of another topic), and then writes the name of each animal on the top lines. The child is then asked to describe the animals.

Therapist: "Tell me about Giraffes".

Child: "A Giraffe is an animal".
"A Giraffe lives in Africa".
"It eats leaves and twigs".
"It has a long neck".

If the child gives one or two word sentences (e.g. Africa, leaves, long neck), the therapist should prompt the child to create whole sentences. As the child gives the list of attributes, the therapist should write each point down on one of the lines directly under the name of the animal.

Therapist: "Good. Now tell me about Chimpanzees".

Child: "A Chimpanzee is an animal."
"A Chimpanzee lives in Africa."
"It eats fruits, nuts, and leaves."
"It is smart."

As the therapist writes down these descriptions, she can line up the similar points for both animals. Next, the therapist should show the child that the chimpanzee and giraffe are both 1) animals and 2) live in Africa. All items that the two topics have in common should be rewritten into the middle part of the diagram.

Finally, the therapist should ask the child to tell her how a _giraffe_ and _chimpanzee_ are the same. The child should be prompted to answer with "They BOTH are animals", or They BOTH eat leaves", etc. _Note: Once the child has a firm grasp of the concept "Same", the therapist can ask the child to tell her how a _giraffe_ and _chimpanzee_, for example, are different. The child can the choose the details that have not been circled._

Why Do Comparisons?

Comparisons are a good way to teach the child to understand the critical information given to him/her in the paragraphs. A piece of information becomes relevant when it is differentiated or when it shares something in common. To illustrate, a lion and a tiger are both cats. However, they are found in different parts of the world and have different markings. The goal is for the child to see connections between types of animals and become more interested in the animal kingdom as a whole (or any other subject that is outwardly focused).

Making Comparisons

The Venn Diagram Comparison exercise gives a visual representation of the concept of same and different. The first time the child does this exercise, the therapist should have all the descriptors of each animal listed. The therapist should direct the child to circle the descriptors that are the same for each animal. Then the therapist can draw an arrow into the middle (while the child observes) and write the common descriptor that the child has just circled in the intersecting circle.

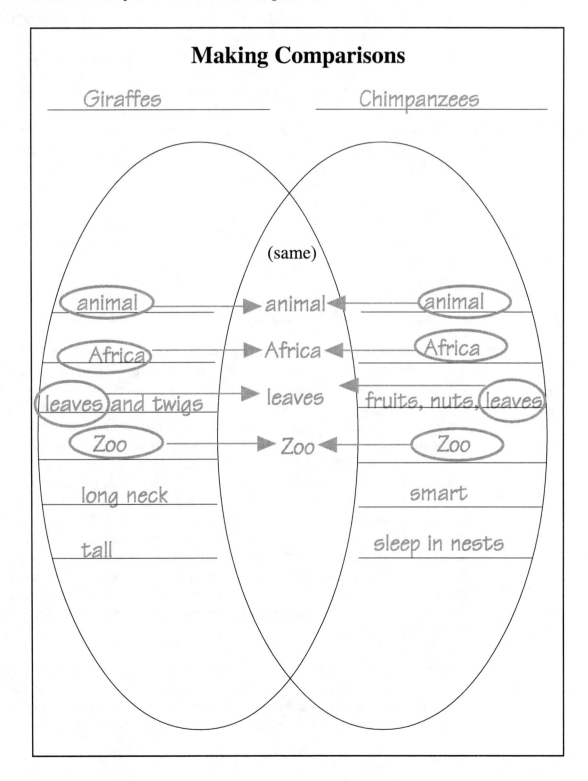

Comparisons (Intermediate & Advanced)

Grid Comparisons

This drill is simply an elaboration of the easier grids used for animals and occupations. It allows the child to give more critical information about two subjects (one at a time) to the therapist. In addition to learning about where the animal lives, what it eats, what it has and what kind of animal it is, the child can also provide information from the paragraphs about whether it lays eggs, and in what part of the world the animal is found. If the child is interested in a particular characteristic of animals that is not "critical", this information can still be added since there is enough room and it will create added interest.

Once the therapist has instructed the child to complete the grid (in much the same way as with the easier grid), then the child is to circle the features that are the same for each animal. For example, if the two animals chosen are lions and monkeys, the characteristic they share is that they both live in Africa. The child should circle the word "Africa" in both columns. In addition, the therapist should have the child describe the animal in full sentences using the information in the grid. Grid comparisons can be made for any subject. We have included a sample of a grid comparison for sports to show the reader the versatility of the grid.

+/- Comparisons (Using True, False and Both)

First, the therapist prepares the drill by writing 10 facts in the column under facts. These facts relate to information taken from the previously introduced paragraphs. To use this drill with animals, the therapist could use these 10 facts on animals e.g. lives in Asia, eats meat, lays eggs, lives in or near water, has black and white stripes, is a mammal, uses tools, lives in groups, sleeps at night, and is cold blooded . Next, the therapist chooses two animals and writes the name of each animal in the two top boxes. Then, the child reads the fact and either places a "+" or "-" directly under the animal, parallel with the relevant fact. The "+" symbol is used when the statement is true, and the "-" symbol is used when the statement is false. The child must circle the "+" or true features that are the same for each animal. The therapist should show the child what to do using the first few facts. Once the child understands the structure of the exercise, s/he should be able to go through the list and evaluate each fact by him/herself. This exercise is a variation of the grid comparison except that more information about the subject is included, and this grid makes it easier for the child to see similarities and differences at a glance. The following examples of +/- comparisons use the topics of occupations and sports, but can be adapted to any topic.

Another variation on this exercise uses the concept of "Both". Instead of using a "+" or "-", the child must indicate whether the facts apply to both subjects being compared, and if not, for which subject the statement is true. The example given on the following page uses sports; however, this exercise is versatile and can be applied to whichever topic is taught.

General Comparisons

Once the child understands the comparisons using animals and occupations and can talk about similarities and differences using the information taught in the paragraphs, it is time to apply this drill to general categories that have not been taught in depth. The purpose of this drill is to teach the child to create original thoughts about similarities and differences. To illustrate, using the General Comparison sheet, the therapist will have the child compare a doll and legos. The child will be asked, "How are a doll and legos the same?". The child will be required to find something similar about these two items such as, "You play with a doll and you play with legos". Then the therapist will ask, "How are a doll and legos different?". The child will answer something like, "A doll can sit but legos can make a tower". Whatever the child says that is remotely correct should be accepted at first. The therapist may have to prompt to improve the structure of the sentence; however, the major goal of this exercise when it is first introduced is for the child to understand the concept of "same and different" in this form and be able to come up with similarities and differences on his/her own. At first, heavy prompting may be necessary; however, it is CRUCIAL that the therapist fade out the prompts very quickly. If the child has difficulty with this concept, cue cards with "they both are", "they both have", "they both use", "they both need", "they both feel" may be used. The "General Comparisons (2)" sheet is simply a more difficult form of the "General Comparison (1)" sheet.

Problems:
Some children have a difficult time learning the concepts of "same" and "different". To help the child understand the concept first visually and then auditorially, the therapist can use a wipe board and illustrate the concepts of same and different, as below:

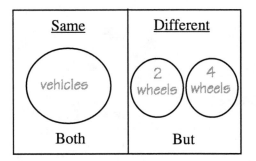

The therapist can say, "Tell me, how are <u>car</u> and <u>bike</u> same?" The therapist can then prompt the child by pointing to "Same" and "Both". The child can then answer, "both vehicles." Then the therapist can ask, "How are a car and bike different?" The therapist can prompt the child by pointing to "Different". The child can answer, "a car has 4 wheels, <u>but</u> a bike as 2 wheels."

Animal Grid Comparison

This exercise is an elaboration of the easier animal comparison. It is introduced to the child in much the same way as the easier grid. The Animal Grid Fill-In sheet should be introduced to the child once s/he has learned two animals from the medium or difficult paragraphs.

Animal **Comparison**

Fill in the grid for each ____ animal ____
Then circle the features that are the same for each ____ animal ____

Feature Compared	Duck	Giraffe
What kind of animal	bird	mammal
Where it lives	In or near water	Africa
What it eats	plants and small animals	leaves and twigs
What it looks like	feathers, beak	4 legs, long brown and yellow neck
How it has babies	lay eggs	baby giraffes
How it sleeps	makes a nest	standing up

Sport Grid Comparison

The Sport Grid Comparison exercise is introduced to the child in much the same way as the earlier Grid Fill-Ins. The Sport Grid Fill-In sheet should be introduced to the child once s/he has learned two sports.

Sport **Comparison**

Fill in the grid for each _____ sport _____
Then circle the features that are the same for each _____ sport _____

Feature Compared	Basketball	Baseball
Kind of Sport: Team or Individual	(Team)	(Team)
Where played?	on a court	on a field
What you need	ball, hoop	ball, bat, bases, glove
Number of Players on each team	5	9
Scoring Unit	baskets	runs
How you score	make a basket	get to home plate

+/- Occupation Comparison

This exercise is an elaboration of the easier occupation comparisons. It is introduced to the child in much the same way as the easy Occupation Grid was taught. The Occupation Grid Fill-In sheet should be used once the child has learned about two occupations from the medium or difficult paragraphs.

+/- Comparison

Look at each _occupation_ fact.
Put a "+" in the box under the correct _occupation_ for each true fact.
Put a "-" in the box under the correct _occupation_ for each fact that is false.
Then circle the "+" or true features that are the same for each _occupation_.

Fact	Chefs	Authors
cooks food	+	−
a man or a lady	+	+
works in a hotel or restaurant	+	−
works with a computer	−	+
wears a white hat or apron	+	−
writes books, stories or poems	−	+
works in an office or at home	−	+
follows a recipe	+	−

+/- Sport Comparison

This exercise is introduced to the child in the same way as the +/- Occupation Comparison. The Sport Grid Fill-In sheet should be used once the child has learned two sports.

+/- Comparison

Look at each ___sport___ fact.
Put a "+" in the box under the correct ___sport___ for each true fact.
Put a "-" in the box under the correct ___sport___ for each fact that is false.
Then circle the "+" or true features that are the same for each ___sport___.

Fact	Baseball	Basketball
team sport	+	+
played on a field	+	-
played with a ball	+	+
score by making a basket	-	+
five players on each team	-	+
you dribble or bounce the ball	-	+
when there are 3 outs, the teams change places	+	-
teams try to make a touchdown	-	-

Sport Comparisons Using "Both"

This exercise should accompany the topic of sports and should be given to the child after s/he has learned about two sports (from the sport paragraphs). The exercise helps reinforce what has been learned and maintains the role of the word "both", thereby widening the type of comparison the child can make. The Sport Comparison exercise illustrates the way to customize an exercise for a specific area of interest. The same structure can be used for different types of interests e.g. dance, gymnastics, musical instruments, art.

Sport Comparisons Using the Concept of Both

Tell which sport _basketball, baseball or Both_ goes with each of the following:

What	Which Sport
score points	basketball
9 players on a team	baseball
game played between 2 teams	both
the San Francisco Giants play this	baseball
score runs	baseball
team sport	both

General Comparisons (1)

This comparison exercise is more difficult than the previous comparison exercises because the child must find similarities and differences without being directed by the structure of the exercise. There are many correct answers to this exercise which gives the child the opportunity to be successful. Once the child understands this exercise well, then it is important to point out the most obvious answers to the child (even if the child correctly gives another answer).

General Comparisons (1)

How are a<u>n apple</u> and <u>a watermelon</u> the same?

They both...
<u>are fruit</u>

How are a<u>n apple</u> and <u>a watermelon</u> different?

A<u>n apple can be red, green, or yellow</u>

But

A <u>watermelon is green.</u>

How are a<u>n ice-cream</u> and <u>cake</u> the same?

They both...
<u>are sweet</u>

How are a<u>n ice-cream</u> and <u>cake</u> different?

A <u>an ice-cream is cold</u>

But

A <u>cake is not cold.</u>

General Comparisons (2)

Prerequisite: The child should be able to complete a grid comparison before this General Comparison sheet is introduced.

This comparison exercise is much harder than the first general comparison exercise because the child must find as many similarities and differences as s/he can. This exercise is worth doing over a period of years because it works on the child's logical and critical thinking skills. Once the child is comfortable with general comparisons, this sheet should be removed. At this point, the child should be able to compare two subjects without using any visual prompts.

General Comparisons (2)

Look at this comparison form.
Answer the questions below.

How _____ are chefs and authors _____ the same?

They Both...

_____ can be a man or a lady _____

_____

_____

_____

_____

How _____ are chefs and authors _____ different?

Author writes books, stories, or poems

An author works in an office and a chef works in a restaurant or hotel.

An author types on the computer and a chef uses a stove and oven.

A chef wears a white hat or an apron.

Authors write on paper and do rewrites.

Concluding Remarks About General Knowledge

How To Make This Relevant To Life

Every child has many different topics that are relevant to his/her life. Clearly there are more subjects directly relevant to the child than what is presented in this book. This is why we have attempted to present a method by which to teach the child relevant information, rather than including hundreds of paragraphs that may or may not be relevant. Once parents, therapists, and children are comfortable with this technique of teaching general knowledge, it is important that those who work with the child create paragraphs which are directly relevant to the child and teach him/her pertinent information. This is why the flexibility of this method is so important. As long as the therapist or parent can find the structure of each topic, the child can learn about that topic. Examples of topics that may need to be structured for the child include: holidays and celebrations, sports, recreational activities, hobbies, events, academic subjects.

What's Next In Terms of General Information

After the child has completed all the drills presented in this chapter and used all the materials provided, it <u>may</u> be time to progress to "off the shelf" commercially available materials. These materials must be used in conjunction with the same drills the child has used to this point. The drills should be used until such time as the child can extract the information independently from age appropriate or simple books. This may take years. It is important that the child be able to comprehend the paragraphs included in this book before introducing these books. Even information presented in the easiest books will be too difficult to comprehend without going through all the prepared paragraphs first. For a list of books to use to create paragraphs much like the ones presented in this book, please see the introduction to this chapter.

An additional tool to maintain general knowledge learned through paragraphs are the many workbooks available at teacher supply stores. Some of these workbooks cover much of the academic information the child will be required to know. It is important to introduce workbooks that require a slightly lower ability than that of the child. S/he will then be able to work through the book easily and continue to the next book which will be at the child's skill level. By introducing workbooks, parents and therapists train the child to feel comfortable and competent working independently, which is required in a mainstream classroom.

4

Grammar & Syntax

Introduction to Grammar & Syntax

Pronouns

- Pronoun Classification
- Exercises
- Pronoun Referents
- Exercises

Verbs

- Verb Game and Cards
- Talking about Verbs
- Examples

Nouns

- Noun Game and Cards

WH Questions

- Personal Information
- Question Script
- Where Questions
- Why Questions
- When Questions
- Assorted Topical Questions
- Social Questions
- WH Game and Cards

Super Sentences

- Exercises

Phrase Identification

- Exercises

Parts of Language

- Examples

Grammar and Syntax

The purpose of this chapter is to focus on the certain parts of language that the child has problems with and, through the drills presented, minimize or eliminate the problem. This chapter is not designed to teach the child English grammar.

The first drills introduced work on pronouns, an area typically difficult for children with Autism and other developmental disorders. These drills should be performed many times until the child understands the concept. At first, the child's answers must be heavily prompted in order for the child to understand the structure of the drill. After a while, many children should be able to do these sheets on their own.

We also include exercises to work on nouns and verbs along with a couple of games that are very effective in teaching correct noun and verb usage.

In addition, this chapter focuses on a variety of "WH" questions, including the very basic and the more complex (which need to be customized to the child's knowledge base). We also include a two level "WH" game designed to work on asking and answering "WH" questions.

At the end of the chapter, there are three exercises provided to work on grammar and syntax. The first exercise teaches the child to put together a long sentence (referred to as a super sentence). The Phrase Identification exercise in this chapter has the child categorize phrases based on their function. The most advanced exercise has an older child go through a paragraph and identify the various parts of the language, and thereby, further clarify the various component parts of a sentence.

Why Teach Grammar & Syntax This Way?

Many of the techniques used are similar to the way English as a second language is taught. Although normally developing children do not acquire language in this way, it may be easier for children with language difficulties to learn their primary language as if it were a second language. The idea is to make the rules and structure of language explicit.

How To Teach Pronoun Classification

Prerequisite: Before the child is taught how to classify pronouns s/he should be able to categorize people, places, animals, and things.

The therapist should begin this activity by having the child differentiate between the HE and SHE pronouns only (cross out the columns for IT, WE and THEY).

The therapist first lists 4 to 5 male nouns and pronouns and 4-5 female nouns and pronouns, including familiar proper names such as Billy, Susie, and simple common nouns such as the boy, the girl, the woman, the man, dad, mom, etc.

Then each of the people words must be worked verbally with the child e.g. "Boy. A boy is a _(he)_ " Then, the therapist directs the child to write the word "boy" under HE in the column provided. She should continue through all listed items. For proper names, the therapist should verbally have the child identify the gender e.g. "Billy. Billy is a _(boy)_." A boy is a HE. So Billy is a HE." The therapist should try to lead the child through this reasoning process.

After classifying each of the words, the child should use the target word and corresponding word in a contingent sentence pair e.g. the _boy_ ran to school. _He_ was late. This allows the therapist to see if the child truly understands how the two words relate. The therapist should model this the first time.

Then the singular form for places, animals, and things corresponding to the pronoun IT should be gradually added and mixed with the HE and SHE nouns above.

The therapist should continue this drill, expanding the field to include nouns referring to WE, and THEY. Noun pairs reflecting WE will always include I and another person. THEY can refer to the plural form for people, places, animals, or things. This pronoun will potentially give the child problems at first. For example, a pair such as THE BOY AND THE GIRL is correctly referred to as THEY; however, the child may initially want to place the pair in either the HE or SHE category. The therapist should continue the drill in the same way as above for the object pronouns ME, YOU, HIM, HER, IT and their plural forms US, YOU, and THEM.
EXAMPLES:

<u>we</u>	<u>they</u>	<u>him</u>	<u>her</u>	<u>us</u>
The teacher and I	the girls	the man	the girl	Joe and I
My friend and I	four animals	Mr. Jones	Beth	My family and I
Sue and I	Susie and Billy			

Why Teach Pronoun Classification?

For the child to 1) understand what s/he reads (not simply decode words and sentences), and 2) fully comprehend daily speech, it is important that the child understand the relationship between nouns and pronouns since they are used heavily in even the lowest level of speech. Pronoun reversal is quite common among these children; proper use of pronouns typically must be taught formally in order to have them use pronouns correctly. This drill is the first step after teaching about simple pronoun use i.e. teaching the difference between "I" and "You". Once the child can understand the relationship between pronouns and nouns, then s/he can be introduced to them in sentences (see the Pronoun Referent activity which follows).

Classifying Pronouns

This exercise teaches the child to classify pronouns. This skill is important for reading comprehension. The child should write each word under the appropriate pronoun.

Classifying Pronouns

Write each word or phrase in the correct pronoun box.

Words: boy, dog, the girls, you and I, tree, girl

he	she	it	we	they
boy	girl	dog tree	you and I	the girls

How To Teach Pronoun Referents

Prerequisite: The child should be able to classify familiar people, places, animals, and things into the categories of 1) I, You, He, She or It (singular subject pronouns), and 2) We, You, and They (plural subject pronouns). S/he should also be able to classify familiar people, places, animals and things into the categories of 1) Me, You, Him, Her, It (singular object pronouns) and 2) Us, You, Them (plural object pronouns). The pronoun classification activity is a good way to teach this.

NOTE: In previous early language tasks where the child is asked to describe the picture, s/he should have already been exposed to pronoun usage e.g. "Look at the girl. Tell me what she is doing." ----> "She is jumping rope." The classification activity simply expands the child's knowledge and repertoire of pronouns.

To teach pronoun referents in context, the therapist should begin with simple contingent sentences. For example: The boy went to the park. <u>He</u> played in the sand. The pronoun should be underlined. The child should then be directed to circle the word in the previous sentence to which the pronoun refers. The therapist should work through this task verbally with the child: "HE is the pronoun. HE is talking about the <u>(boy)</u>." The child should then draw an arrow from the pronoun to the subject to which it refers.

At first, the therapist should not include more than one pronoun or referent per sentence pair. It is important to make the sentence choices relevant to the child, using names, events, activities that the child is familiar with. Gradually, the therapist can add two subjects and two pronouns, expanding the subjects from including just people to including people, places, and things. As the child masters this activity, the therapist should gradually continue to build and add object pronouns. The number of sentences the child has to analyze should increase, building gradually. Eventually, the child should be required to identify pronouns and their referents in an entire short story. At this point, the therapist can use the story to check reading comprehension.

Why Teach Pronoun Referents In This Way?

Children with language delays often have difficulty in understanding the role and relevance of pronouns in language. In fact, many of them reverse their pronouns and must be taught to use pronouns correctly. The concentration on pronouns will further enhance the child's understanding of the use of pronouns in language. This skill is not only important in everyday speech, but plays an important role in reading comprehension. If the child does not understand pronouns, it is difficult to expect him/her to fully understand what s/he is reading.

Pronoun Referents Exercise

This exercise teaches the child about the relationship between pronouns and nouns. If the child does not understand the role of pronouns, it will be very difficult for him/her to comprehend text and will hamper comprehension of simple conversation.

Pronoun Referents Exercise

A PRONOUN takes the place of a noun.
Circle the noun or nouns that the underlined pronoun refers to. Draw an arrow from the pronoun to its referent.

1. Sue was making her lunch. Her mother said, "Don't forget to put it in your lunch box".

2. The ball rolled into the street. Mike said, "Go get it". Jim said, "No way! I'm not gonna".

3. The kids went to the movie. Sue said, "It was really good". Jane said, "Yeah, I think so too".

4. Jim and Mike went to a party. They had a good time and told their mom that it was fun.

5. Carly said, "I want a turn on the swing". Stacey said, "No, you already played on it for a long time."

How To Play the Verb Game

The verb game begins with the therapist taking a card from the top of the pile and adding a verb to it. For example, if the therapist chose "_____ the ball", she could say: "Kick the ball". Then it would be the child's turn. He could say: "Throw the ball". Then the therapist would turn the card toward herself and say: "Catch the Ball". Then she would turn it back toward the child and the child could say: "Roll the Ball". The back and forth should continue for approximately four turns per card (more turns as the child learns more verbs). Eventually, the child will come to memorize the various verbs that go with the nouns on the card. The child should be shown any verb that is new to the child e.g. if the child does not know what "roll" means, the therapist should take a ball and roll it to show him/her. The therapist should be as creative as possible after "typical" responses to complete each phrase are provided e.g. stand on the ball, sit on the ball, hide the ball. The purpose is to encourage the child to be as creative as possible with his/her verb choices. The more people who play this game with the child the better, since they will expose the child to more verbs.

Once the child has learned these 24 cards and all the possible verb choices, the therapist can create more. The new verbs should be age appropriate and relevant to the child.

What's the Purpose of the Verb Game?

This game is intended for the child who has difficulty accessing and varying verbs during story telling and general conversational activities. The purpose of this activity is to increase the number of verbs the child uses with familiar nouns.

Game Cards For Verb Game

These are reproducible game cards to be used as explained on the previous page. They can be photocopied onto card stock to ensure their durability.

_____ the ball	_____ the apple
_____ the bed	_____ the book
_____ the slide	_____ the car
_____ the cup	_____ the T.V.

Game Cards For Verb Game

These are reproducible game cards to be used as explained on the previous page. They can be photo-copied onto card stock to ensure their durability.

_____ the park	_____ the bread
_____ the paper	_____ the milk
_____ your hands	_____ the cake
_____ the pool	_____ the bike

Game Cards For Verb Game

These are reproducible game cards to be used as explained on the previous page. They can be photocopied onto card stock to ensure their durability.

_____ the baby

_____ the water

_____ the video

_____ the chair

_____ the girl

_____ the music

_____ the boy

_____ the grass

How To Talk About Verbs

The child who has difficulties finding verbs may be helped by verb lists. First, the verbs should be presented to the child on a blackboard or large sheet of paper so it is easier at a glance for the child to find the verb s/he needs. Then, the topic that relates to the verbs should be discussed. The child and therapist should take turns making action statements about the topic, such as "I like to swim at the beach". If the topic is the beach, then all the obvious relevant verbs for the beach should be provided. After a while, the child will memorize which verbs go with which topics and the therapist should fade the verb lists.

Note: The lists presented in this book are in present tense; however, if the child has difficulty with past tense, they should be presented in the past tense to address the problem. The same principle applies for future tense. In addition, it is important that the lists on the following page are presented on a black board or large sheet of paper (not as they appear in long vertical lists on the following page since that format will confuse a child).

Example of a Verb List

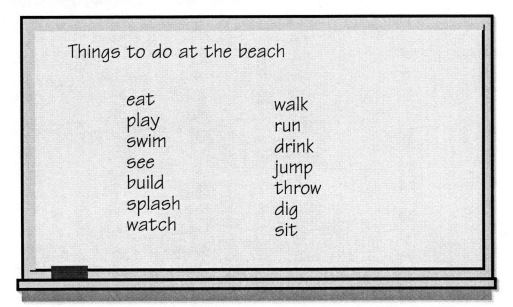

Things to do at the beach

eat	walk
play	run
swim	drink
see	jump
build	throw
splash	dig
watch	sit

Why Teach Verbs In This Way?

This is another example of a visual prompt that allows the child to communicate better about a particular subject. By giving the child a list of verbs, the dialogue will be easier for him/her and s/he will experience more success. In addition, the child will come to memorize verbs that typically fit into particular settings and it will be easier for him to spontaneously verbalize about those settings when not working with a therapist.

Examples of Other Verb Subjects

The verbs listed below have been presented so the therapist can choose from a number of topics to work on with the child. The therapist should create a verb list about any topic of interest to the child to, thereby, introduce appropriate verbs into the setting. When making up a verb list, it is important the therapist use verbs that are simple and have meaning to the child. If the child does not know what a verb means, the therapist should demonstrate the verb before using it in a verb list. It is also important that the verb lists be presented in large letters on a blackboard or a large sheet of paper so the child can read the verb easily at a glance. In the beginning, it is a good idea to use only a few verbs at once. As the child becomes more comfortable using a few verbs, more verbs can be added.

Things To Do...

... at school	... at the zoo	... in the kitchen	... to get ready for bed	... at the park	... at a party
read	see	eat	brush	play	play
play	feed	cook	comb	ride	open
write	watch	bake	wash	dig	blow
see	eat	fry	shampoo	see	see
eat	drink	boil	floss	eat	eat
listen	buy	make	undress	swing	sing
sing	give	mix	bathe	walk	dance
count	laugh at	stir	shower	run	sit
look at	look at	pour	read	climb	give
drink	talk to	cut	hug	drink	drink
color		chop	tuck	jump	laugh
talk		beat	sing	throw	smile
draw		knead	rock	kick	
cook		put in	climb	sit	
paint		clean	put on	slide	
make					
run					
sit					
ride					
cut					
glue					

How To Play the Noun Game

The noun game is similar to the verb game. The Noun Game begins with the therapist taking a card off the top of the pile and adding a noun to it. So for example, if the therapist chose "Eat _____ ", she could say, "Eat the hamburger". Then it would be the child's turn. He could say, "Eat the bread". Then the therapist would turn the card toward herself and say, "Eat the pizza". Then she would turn it back toward the child and the child could say, "Eat the ice-cream". The turn taking should continue for approximately four turns per card (more as time progresses). Eventually, the child will come to memorize the various nouns that go together with the verbs. The therapist should introduce any noun that the child does not understand by showing the child a picture of the noun or giving the child an actual item e.g. if the child does not know what a "hat" is, the therapist should take a hat (or a picture of a hat) and show the child. The therapist should be as creative as possible after the child has memorized the "typical" responses to complete each phrase- the purpose is to encourage the child to be creative with his/her noun choices. The more people who do this activity with the child, the more variety in nouns the child will learn since every adult brings original ideas to the exercise.

Once the child has learned these 24 cards and all the obvious noun choices, the therapist can create more. The new ones should be appropriate in age and relevance to the child.

What's the Purpose of the Noun Game

This game is intended for the child who has difficulty accessing and varying nouns during story telling and general conversational activities. The purpose of this activity is to increase the number of nouns the child uses with familiar verbs.

Game Cards For Noun Game

These are reproducible game cards to be used as explained on the previous page. They can be photocopied onto card stock to ensure their durability.

roll _____	**eat** _____
make _____	**read** _____
go _____	**ride** _____
drink _____	**watch** _____

Game Cards For Noun Game

These are reproducible game cards to be used as explained on the previous page. They can be photocopied onto card stock to ensure their durability.

cut ✂

go to _____	**cut** _____
fold _____	**pour**_____
wash _____	**mix** _____
swim _____	**drive** _____

Game Cards For Noun Game

These are reproducible game cards to be used as explained on the previous page. They can be photocopied onto card stock to ensure their durability.

splash _____	pat _____
buy _____	sit in _____
catch _____	listen to _____
tease _____	lay _____

How To Teach WH Questions

Prerequisite: Before the following exercises are introduced, the child must already know how to visually recognize WHAT, WHO, and WHERE in books. For example, when the therapist points to a dog in a book and asks: "What is it", we assume that the child can answer "Dog". The following activities require that the child has mastered simple WH Question visual recognition (as illustrated above).

1. The first activity designed to work on WH Questions provides personal information questions the child should be able to answer. The therapist should work on the list so the child can answer personal information questions, even if only by rote.

2. The next activity is a Question Script designed to teach the child the type of answers WH questions require. This script can be understood best by using examples to illustrate the pattern. For example, if the child is having difficulty with DID WHAT, then the therapist should demonstrate this concept by going back to a picture (in a children's book) and asking the child, "What is the girl doing?", getting the answer from the child and then closing the book and saying, "The girl did what?". The therapist must then wait for the child to say the action. Initially, some WH questions may be confusing; however, after concentrating on other WH questions and answers, the concepts should become better understood.

3. We have also provided a several lists of WH questions and answers to teach the child. Customizing these lists will help the child understand each concept better because of their relevance to the child and his/her knowledge base.

4. Once the child is familiar with all the different types of WH Questions, they should be mixed. We have included samples of WH Questions that can be used. It is important to create new WH Questions when the child is required to learn something new. This will help him/her grasp the concept, and show the therapist where the weaknesses are in the child's understanding of the newly introduced concept.

Why Teach WH Questions This Way?

Children with language delays often have difficulty with some of the WH Questions. Every child is different and so are the deficits for each child. The generally agreed upon order of difficulty for these children, from easiest to hardest, is: WHAT, WHO, WHERE, WHEN , WHY and HOW. However, many very bright children do not follow this sequence. Therefore, it is best to concentrate on the particular child's weakness rather than follow a conventional order. All the WH questions are designed to relate to the specific child's life and/or knowledge that the child has acquired. It is important that the therapist understand that these are just samples of WH questions the child should know. Every time the child completes a general information module (such as animals, occupations, sports, or planets), WH questions should be designed in the same way as the ones that have been provided in this book. In this way, the child will truly understand the relevance and meaning of the various WH questions, particularly the difficult ones such as WHY and HOW.

Personal Information Questions

The following questions are common social questions that every child is usually required to answer. It is important to choose the questions from the list that are age appropriate e.g. a five year old should know his/her name and age, but should not be required to know what his/her father does for a living).

Personal Information Questions

1. What is your name?
2. How old are you?
3. When is your birthday?
4. What grade are you in?
5. What school do you go to?
6. Who is your teacher?
7. Where do you live?
8. What is your address?
9. What is your phone number?
10. How many people are in your family?
11. Do you have a brother?
12. Do you have a sister?
13. How many sisters do you have?
14. How many brothers do you have?
15. What are their names?
16. How old are they?
17. Do you have a pet?
18. What does your dad do?
19. What does your mom do?
20. What do you like to eat?
21. What do you like to drink?
22. What is your favorite thing to do?
23. Where do you like to go?
24. What do you like to read about?
25. What is your favorite movie?
26. What is your favorite game?
27. What don't you like to do?
28. Who do you play with at school?

Question Script

The following script explains what each question does. This script should be read with the child before working on WH questions. When the child runs into difficulty with the question, the therapist can say, "Remember, WHO is a person" or "WHERE is a place".

All About Questions

A thing answers a WHAT question.

A person answers a WHO questions.

A place answers a WHERE question.

Time answers WHEN questions

An action word or verb answers a DID WHAT question.

Where Questions

These are the very basic answers to WHERE questions that the child should learn. Once the child has learned some of these answers, WHERE questions that naturally occur in the child's environment should be taught. For example, when the parent goes to the gas station, s/he should say, "Where are we?" and help the child say, "At the gas station". Then the parent could add, "We buy gas at the gas station", followed by, "Where do we buy gas?" ... "at the gas station". In this way, WHERE questions and answers become relevant.

Where Questions

1. Where do we find a doctor? ...in a hospital or office.
2. Where do we keep milk? ... in the refrigerator.
3. Where do we learn? ... at school.
4. Where do we go swimming? ... in the swimming pool.
5. Where do we buy food? ... at the grocery store.
6. Where do we see airplanes? ... at the airport.
7. Where do we eat our dinner? ... in the kitchen, at a restaurant, etc.
8. Where do we keep our clothes? ... in the drawer, in the closet.
9. Where do we go out to eat? ... at McDonald's, etc.
10. Where do we see the moon? ... in the sky at night.
11. Where do we keep money? ... in the bank.
12. Where do we see movies? ... at the movie theater.
13. Where do we buy pies, cakes, and bread? ... at the bakery.
14. Where do we get a hair cut? ... at the hair dresser, barber, etc.
15. Where do we buy toys? ... at the toy store.
16. Where do we dig in the sand? ... at the beach.
17. Where do we see a whale? ... at the aquarium.
18. Where do we get our teeth checked? ... at the dentist.

For additional What, Who, Where, When, Why, and How questions, the MEER2 book is available from LinguiSystems, Inc., (800)776-4332.

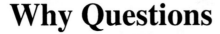

Why Questions

These are the answers to basic WHY questions that the child should learn. This concept is very difficult for some children and may take years to internalize. Answers to these questions will be memorized by the child. The hope is that the child will eventually understand the concept by seeing the pattern and by creating WHY-BECAUSE relationships that are meaningful to the child. The question must be asked in two different ways. The therapist should say, **"We wash our hands because...?"** The child should answer, "because they're dirty". Once the child can answer in this way, then the therapist should ask the question in the following form: **"Why do we wash our hands?"** The child should still give the identical answer.

Why Questions

1. We wash our hands because _they're dirty._

2. We sleep because _we are tired._

3. We wear coats _to keep warm._

4. We go to the doctor because _we feel sick._

5. We go to school to _learn._

6. We eat food because _we are hungry._

7. We drink liquids because _we are thirsty._

8. We need money so that _we can buy things._

9. We need clocks to _tell what time it is._

10. We go to the zoo to _see the animals._

11. We need cars in order to _drive places._

12. We have windows so that _we can see outside._

13. We need eyes so that _we can see._

14. We need ears so that _we can hear._

15. We need a mouth so that _we can taste and eat food._

16. We need a nose so that _we can smell._

17. We wash our clothes because _they are dirty._

18. We brush our teeth so that _they are clean._

19. We get our hair cut because _it is too long._

20. We need lights so that _we can see when it's dark._

When Questions

The list below contains basic WHEN questions that the child should learn. It is important to customize the list to the child since it must be relevant to him/her for the concept to be understood. This list alone is not enough to teach time concepts; it should be augmented with the strategies on teaching time presented in the chapter on Academics and Language Based Concepts.

When Questions

1. I go to school on _____, _____, _____, _____, and _____.

2. I don't go to school on a _____.

3. I work with Sue on _____, _____, _____, _____, and _____.

4. I work with Jim on _____, _____, _____, _____.

6. I don't work with anybody on _____. I have a day off from work on _____.

7. I go to ballet every _____.

8. I go to piano lessons on _____.

9. I carry an umbrella when __*it rains*__.

10. I empty the trash when __*it's full*__.

11. I go to the doctor when __*I am sick*__.

12. I raise my hand to ask a question when __*I don't know*__

13. My dad comes home from work at __*night*__.

14. I go to the grocery store when __*I need to buy food*__.

15. I get my haircut when __*it's too long*__.

16. I go swimming when __*it's hot*__.

17. A fireman comes when __*there's a fire*__.

18. I wash my hands when __*they are dirty*__

Topical Questions Mixed (Animals)

These are samples of the mixed questions designed for the Animal General Knowledge activities in Chapter 3. It is important that the actual questions used relate only to the animals the child has already learned well. The goal of this exercise is not to teach about animals; rather, it is to get the child to answer questions correctly based on knowledge the child has learned as well as maintain the information on animals already learned.

Mixed Topical Animal Questions

1. What does a bird do?
2. Is a cow a mammal or a reptile?
3. What does a lizard eat?
4. Where do alligators live?
5. What cat is the fastest runner?
6. Where do amphibians live?
7. How does a turtle protect itself?
8. Do reptiles have dry or wet skin?
9. What does a rhinoceros have on its head?
10. How many legs does an insect have?
11. Is a ladybug a bird or an insect?
12. What type of animal is an iguana?
13. Do amphibians have dry or wet skin?
14. What do snakes eat?
15. Where do tigers live?
16. Name three mammals.
17. What animal is a chimpanzee like?
18. How does a turtle's shell feel?
19. What animal is called King of the Beasts?
20. Is a snake a reptile or an amphibian?
21. What does a frog jump with?
22. How does a lizard run?
23. What do birds eat?
24. Are alligators dangerous or safe?
25. Is a frog's skin wet or dry?
26. What kind of weather do penguin's like?
27. How many legs does a lizard have?
28. Are amphibians like reptiles or mammals?
29. Is a turtle a mammal or a reptile?
30. Where do birds live?
31. Is a frog a reptile or amphibian?
32. What kind of feet does a turtle have?
33. Are amphibians cold or warmblooded?
34. Is a lizard an amphibian or a reptile?
35. What does a frog use to catch food?
36. What does a turtle hatch from?
37. What kind of weather does a lizard like?
38. What do amphibians have?
39. What helps a bird fly?
40. Why does a turtle hide in its shell?

Topical Questions Mixed (Occupations)

These are samples of the mixed questions designed for the Occupation General Knowledge activities in Chapter 3. It is important that the actual questions used relate only to the occupations the child has already learned well. The goal of this exercise is not to teach about occupations; rather, it is to get the child to answer questions correctly based on knowledge that the child has learned as well as maintain the information on occupations already learned.

Mixed Topical Occupation Questions

1. What does a farmer do?
2. Where does a doctor work?
3. Who uses a cash register?
4. Who works on a farm?
5. What does a doctor use to help him work?
6. Where does a clerk work?
7. Who helps sick people?
8. What does a farmer drive?
9. What does a clerk do?
10. Where does a farmer work?
11. Who helps to keep you healthy?
12. Who do you give your money to in a store?
13. Who grows animals and plants?
14. Where does a fireman work?
15. What are crops?
16. Who uses a mirror to look inside your mouth?
17. Who uses a stethoscope?
18. Who puts your groceries in a bag at the store?
19. What special clothes does a fire fighter wear?
20. What is livestock?
21. Where does a dentist work?
22. What kinds of animals live on a farm?
23. What does a fire fighter use?
24. Who checks for cavities?
25. How does a fire fighter get to a fire?
26. What does a mailman do?
27. Where does a police officer work?
28. Who gives you a menu?
29. Who writes a ticket?
30. What does a mailman use?
31. What does a police officer wear?
32. Where does a waiter work?
33. Who makes sure rules are not broken?
34. Who works in a post office?
35. What does a waiter do?
36. Where does a musician work?
37. Who cooks food in a restaurant?
38. What does a carpenter do?
39. Who writes books and stories?
40. What does a chef use?
41. Who uses tools to build?
42. Who plays musical instruments.
43. Where does a chef work?
44. What does a chef do?
45. What does an author do?

Occupations:
farmer
doctor
dentist
clerk
fire fighter
police officer
waiter
mailman
musician
author
chef
carpenter
teacher
librarian
engineer

Sports: Mixed Questions

These are samples of the mixed questions designed for the Sports General Knowledge activities in Chapter 3. It is important that the actual questions used relate only to the sports the child has already learned well. This is an example of how mixed topical questions can be customized to a particular child's interest. General knowledge about sports need not be taught to all children. Children who are going to have many social opportunities that revolve around sports, should learn about sports.

Mixed Topical Sports Questions

Basketball

1. Is basketball a team or individual sport?
2. Where do you play basketball?
3. What do you need to play basketball?
4. How many teams play in a basketball game?
5. How many players are on each team?
6. What can you do with a basketball?
7. Where do you try to shoot a basketball?
8. What does a hoop have?
9. How many points is each basket worth?
10. Which team wins a basketball game?
11. What is the name of the NBA basketball team in our area?

Baseball

1. Is baseball an individual or team sport?
2. Where do you play baseball?
3. What do you need to play baseball?
4. How many teams play in a baseball game?
5. How many players are on each baseball team?
6. What does the hitting or batting team in baseball try to do?
7. What does the catching team do?
8. How many outs does the hitting team get?
9. When do the hitting and fielding teams change places?
10. How does a team score a run?
11. Which team wins a baseball game?
12. What are the names of the 2 major league baseball teams?

Football

1. Is football an individual or team sport?
2. Where do you play football?
3. What do you need to play football?
4. How many teams play in a football game?
5. How many players are on the field for each team?
6. What can a player do with a football?
7. How many units or groups of players does a football team have?
8. What are the two units called?
9. What does the Offensive Unit try to do?
10. What does the Defensive Unit try to do?
11. How does a team score points in a football game?
12. Which team wins a football game?
13. What is the name of the pro football team from San Francisco?

Mixed WH-Questions (Baseball Diagram)

These are samples of the mixed questions designed to be used with a Baseball Field Diagram. These questions must be asked using a diagram so the child can use the visual prompt to answer the questions. This is particularly useful if the child is to be expected to play the game. This format can be adapted to any sport the child needs to know.

Mixed WH-Questions for Baseball Diagram

1. What is this called?
2. Where is the outfield?
3. Where is the infield?
4. Where is the hitting/batting team?
5. How many players are on the hitting/batting team? (have the child point to and count)
6. Where is the fielding/catching team?
7. How many players are on the fielding team? (have the child point to and count)
8. How many players play in the outfield? (point and count)
9. How many players play in the infield? (point and count)
10. Where is 1st/2nd/3rd base/home plate?
11. Which player is going to hit/bat the ball? What is he called?
12. Which player is going to throw/pitch the ball? What is he called?
13. Which player plays 1st base? 2nd base? 3rd base? (point to)
14. Which player plays between 2nd and 3rd base? (point to)
15. Who sits behind home plate? What does he do? What does he wear? Why?
16. Who stands behind the catcher? What does he do?
17. Which player plays in left field? center field? right field?
18. Where does the batter run when he hits the ball?
19. Show me where the batter runs when he hits a single.
20. Show me where the batter runs when he hits a double.
21. Show me where the batter runs when he hits a triple.
22. Show me where the batter runs when he hits a home run.
23. How does a player on the hitting team score a run?

Social Questions

These are samples of mixed social questions designed to be used as conversation openers. The child should be taught to answer as well as ask these questions. For more information on how to teach questions, please refer to the Comment-Question drills in the Social Language Chapter.

Social Questions

Questions About Places

Where did you go _____? (weekend, last night, yesterday)

What did you do at _____?

Who did you go with?

Did you have a good time?

When did you go?

What did you do there?

Questions About Things

What's your favorite _____?

What _____ do you like?

Do you have _____?

What kind of _____ do you have?

Where did you get _____?

When did you get _____?

Who gave you _____?

Do you like _____?

Questions About Doing Things

Do you like to _____?

Where do you play _____?

Who do you play _____ with?

When did you play _____?

What's your favorite _____ to do? (or play)

How To Play The WH Question Game

To play the WH QUESTIONS GAME, the therapist must create the spinner like the one shown on the following page (a spinner taken from another game can be adapted to look like the spinner shown). The first time the game is played, the therapist chooses a topic that the child knows a lot about and enjoys talking about e.g. Disneyland. Then she spins the spinner and asks a question based on the question type indicated by the spinner. For example, if the spinner pointed to "What", she could ask the child, "What do you like to do at Disneyland?" The child is then required to answer. Next, it is the child's turn. Let's say s/he spins the spinner and it lands on "Where". S/he could ask, "Where is Disneyland?" The therapist would then answer, "Los Angeles", or "Anaheim" depending on the age and sophistication of the child. The topic of Disneyland could be used for as many spins as there is interest. Once that subject is exhausted, the child has the opportunity to choose a new subject.

Once the child thoroughly understands the game and has played it many times without too much difficulty (based on the easy and relevant topics chosen by the therapist and the child), then it is time to make the game slightly more difficult by constraining the topics. This is where the list of topics (in card form) can be used. When playing with cards, they should be stacked in a pile. The child must pick a card and is required to spin. The child must ask a question based on the topic card chosen and the WH question type the spinner lands upon. Then it is the therapist's turn. She chooses a card and spins the spinner. The game proceeds with the therapist and child taking turns as described above.

Once the child becomes good at the game, the therapist can make the game more difficult by using the more difficult spinner. This second spinner mixes HOW and WHICH questions with other easy questions (if the child lands on the ?, s/he has a free choice of question type).

NOTE: This is a good game to use with peers or siblings to work on both socialization and language.

Why Teach WH Questions This Way?

This game is designed to promote the child's use of mixed questions. The game constrains the conversation so that the child must use a variety of questions that s/he may otherwise not use. Most children with language delays do not ask many different questions. We hope that the child will learn to ask many different types of questions and generalize the question types from the game to unstructured situations in life. We use a game with topics that are interesting to the child so that practicing questions will not seem as tedious for the child.

WH Question Game - Easy

The WH game is designed to get the child to ask and answer questions. For example, when the spinner lands on "What", the child must ask a question about the topic that begins with "What". The easy version of this game uses the What, Who, Where and When WH questions. The more difficult versions adds two more difficult WH questions. It is a good idea to make sure the child can easily answer the first set of WH questions before progressing to the harder set. "How Many" and "Which" can be used in both the easy and more difficult versions.

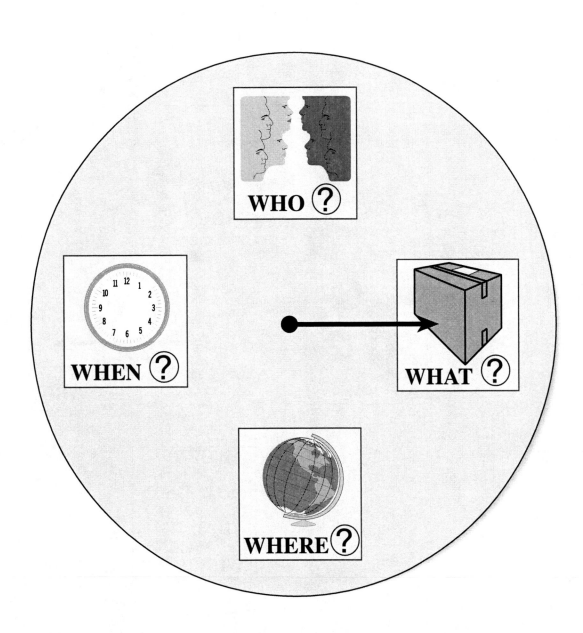

WH Question Game - Difficult

This is the more difficult version of WH game designed to get the child to ask and answer questions. It is a good idea to make sure the child can easily answer the first set of WH questions before going on to this harder set. For this set, when the spinner lands on "Which", for example, the child must ask a question about the topic that begins with "Which". The difficult version of this game uses the Which, How, and How Many WH questions. In addition, a wild card is available on the bottom. When the child lands on the wild card, s/he can choose any WH question s/he pleases (from either the easy or difficult set). "Why" can be added to the WH Question Game; however, it is a very difficult "WH" question to incorporate into the game and should be used only when the child understands "Why/Because" well.

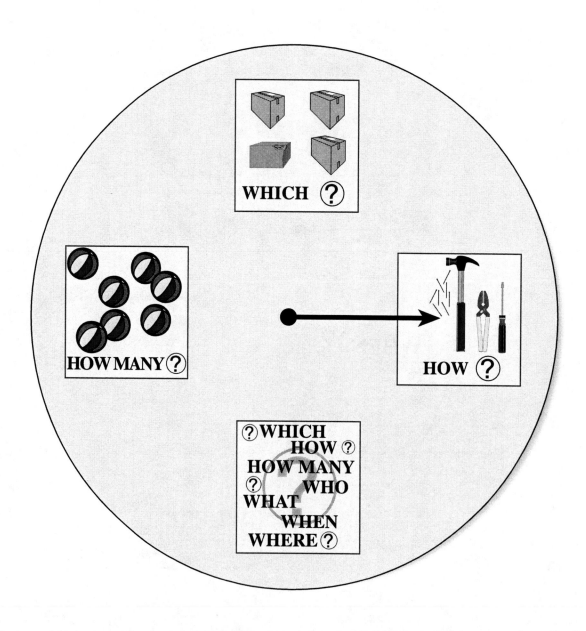

Game Cards For WH Game

These are reproducible game cards to be used as explained on the previous page. They can be photocopied onto card stock to ensure their durability. Any topics relevant to the child should be added.

swimming	**holidays**
favorite book	**the park**
what makes you happy	**birthdays**
a computer game	**what makes you sad**

Game Cards For WH Game

These are reproducible game cards to be used as explained on the previous pages. They can be photocopied onto card stock to ensure their durability.

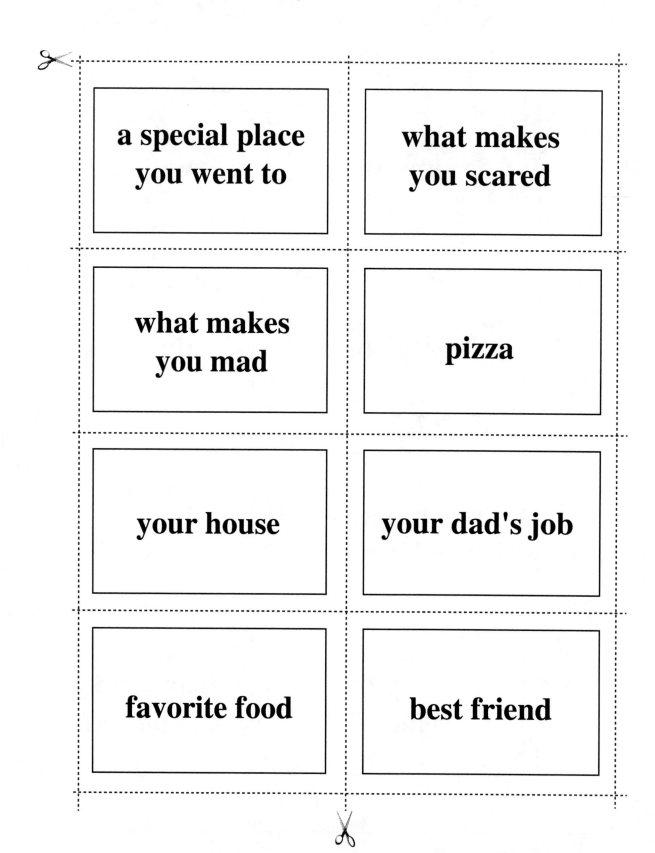

a special place you went to	**what makes you scared**
what makes you mad	**pizza**
your house	**your dad's job**
favorite food	**best friend**

Game Cards For WH Game

These are reproducible game cards to be used as explained on the previous pages They can be photocopied onto card stock to ensure their durability.

roller skating	**a problem**
family	**favorite game**
the beach	**your grandma**
school	**last night**

Game Cards For WH Game

These are reproducible game cards to be used as explained on the previous pages. They can be photocopied onto card stock to ensure their durability.

yesterday	**favorite pet**
shopping	**something dangerous**
the mall	**Disneyland**
your room	**favorite T.V. show**

Game Cards For WH Game

These are reproducible game cards to be used as explained on the previous pages. They can be photocopied onto card stock to ensure their durability.

favorite sport	**thanksgiving**
baseball	**basketball**
vacation	**football**
animal	**cartoon character**

Game Cards For WH Game

These are reproducible game cards to be used as explained on the previous pages. They can be photocopied onto card stock to ensure their durability.

something fun	**barbie dolls**
being proud	**bugs**
favorite place to go	**trains**
riding bikes	**coins**

How To Teach Language With Super Sentences

This popular activity can be found in many workbooks designed for children with language delays. The forms on the following page show PRESENT, PAST and FUTURE tenses; however, when teaching super sentences, it is important to teach each type separately. The child should learn the present tense first and should only be introduced to the past tense when the present tense is well understood. After the past tense is solid, then the child should learn the future tense. On each sheet in the appendix, there are three super sentences. It is a good idea to do at least three sentences in one session for the child to understand the pattern. The therapist should begin by modeling how he/she makes a super sentence. Then s/he should start getting the child involved by asking him/her questions about the subject. So, for example, if the therapist chooses a MAN, she should write it in the "who or what?" box. Then she should say, "Tell me about the man" and "Describe the man". Then the child should give an answer (e.g. tall, short, nice) and the therapist should write it on the form. The therapist should continue prompting the child until each box is complete. Once a sentence has been created, the child should read it aloud. Then the therapist should ask questions regarding the sentence e.g. "When did the dog jump in the yard?", "Where did he jump?", or "What did the dog do?"

Why Teach Using Super Sentences?

The idea behind Super Sentences is to show the child the structure of a sentence. Often, children with autism and related disorders respond very positively to structure; therefore, if the child begins to understand the structure of all sentences of this type it is easier for him/her to 1) understand the meaning of the sentence, 2) be able to answer questions, and 3) know the appropriate order of the different components that comprise a sentence. Of course, there are many complex sentences that do not fit the above format. This sentence structure, however, is very common in the English language and can be used as a crutch.

Super Sentences

This exercise teaches children the parts of a sentence and gives them the opportunity to create their own sentence in a structured way. The goal of this exercise is for the child to start to understand the function of each part of the sentence so s/he will be able to understand and create longer sentences.

Note: Past, Present and Future are on the same sheet to show how each form should be completed; however, when the child is introduced to the drill, it is **VERY IMPORTANT** to introduce each verb tense separately. They should not be mixed until the child has a firm grasp of each tense.

Building a Sentence

Fill in the boxes with words to make a long sentence.

Present Tense

	describing words	who or what?	does what?	where?	when?
The	brown	dog	is jumping	in the yard	at night.

Past Tense

	describing words	who or what?	does what?	where?	when?
The	brown	dog	jumped	in the yard	at night.

Future Tense

	describing words	who or what?	does what?	where?	when?
The	brown	dog	will jump	in the yard	at night.

How To Teach Phrase Identification

The therapist should introduce this drill by asking the child to decide what the phrase is about. For example, the therapist should ask, "Does "the kids" answer a Where question, a When question, a Did What question or a Who question?". Once the child answers, s/he should be able to mark the correct cell on the sheet. At first, the therapist will probably have to heavily prompt the child, helping him/her finish the sheet successfully. Once the child understands what to do, the therapist should fade out the prompts. Eventually, the child should be able to do this drill completely by him/herself without the therapist being in the room.

Once the child can do this drill easily, the therapist should do the same drill orally. The therapist should ask the child without a visual prompt which question the phrase answers. This is VERY difficult and many children will not be able to complete this level of the drill. It is not a necessary stage to reach; however, this drill does work on the child's auditory comprehension.

 PROBLEMS: If the child has great difficulty answering the question, the therapist should simplify the drill by using phrases that answer only one type of question (the question which is the child 's strength). Once the child can answer this one type of question, she should introduce more phrases that answer another type of question. This will show the child different examples of the same type of question. Eventually the therapist should mix the phrases as shown on the example which follows. For example, the therapist should have the child practice Where questions only. Once Where questions are solid, then the therapist should introduce When questions. Eventually, when all the questions have been worked on separately, they can be mixed.

NOTE: This activity is a great activity to follow the Super Sentence drills because the Super Sentence drill teaches the child to compose a sentence using phrases, while the Identifying Phrases drill shows the child what s/he has done.

Why Teach Phrase Identification?

The Phrase identification drill helps teach the structure of the language. Since children with developmental disorders learn faster when they understand the pattern or structure of any concept, it is important to work on their understanding of the structure of sentences. To accomplish this, it is important to understand the concept that a phrase (not just a word) conveys information and that language is composed of a variety of phrases to bring across information. For example, the word "in" tells the reader that an object is in a place; however, "in the bag" tells you exactly where the object is. The word "in", and the words "the bag" must be comprehended together in order for the child to understand the sentence.

Identifying Phrases

This exercise teaches children to identify the various parts of a sentence by their function. This is another way to work on WH questions visually in order to improve the child's auditory understanding.

Identifying Phrases

Read each phrase. Put an X under what each phrase tells about.

	Who/What?	Did What?	Where?	When?
1. the kids	X			
2. earlier today				X
3. bought lunch		X		
4. in the bag			X	
5. Sue's desk	X			
6. under the table			X	
7. rode the bike		X		
8. the baseball coach	X			
9. next to the T.V.			X	
10. before dinner				X

Write a phrase that tells *who or what* ___the girls___.

Write a phrase that tells *did what* ___went swimming___.

Write a phrase that tells *where* ___at the pool___.

Write a phrase that tells *when* ___in the morning___.

How To Teach Parts of Language

This exercise has the child read a paragraph and identify the part of each sentence that s/he has problems with. For example, if the child has difficulty with finding and conjugating verbs, the exercise has the child go through the entire paragraph and circle the verb or verbs in each sentence. After doing several of these paragraphs, the child will become more familiar with verbs, particularly the purpose or role of verbs in a sentence. The role of the therapist is to identify the child's weaknesses within the language and then introduce the appropriate drill. There is no point in doing drills in areas that are not problematic. We provide an example of a paragraph that has been used for each part of the language; however, any paragraph can be used. Keep in mind the child's reading ability - make sure the paragraph is easy for the child to read. The best types of paragraphs to use are those that relate to and are of interest to the child. These paragraphs should be written by either the parent or therapist.

This is quite an advanced exercise and should not be used until the child is proficient in all the easier drills in the grammar and syntax chapter.

Why Teach Parts of Language This Way?

By teaching grammar and syntax through usage, the child develops a better understanding, awareness and knowledge of different word forms. The idea is to go over the patterns several times rather than have the child be able to identify nouns from verbs taken out of context. In addition, by making the examples relevant to each child (by personalizing them), the child has a better opportunity to figure out the structure of the language.

Example - Nouns

The parent or therapist must present the child with a paragraph something like the one below and have the child find all the nouns in the paragraph.

After the (bears) made (porridge) for (breakfast,) they poured it in the (bowls) to cool and went for a (walk.) Then a little (girl) named (Goldilocks) came to the bears' (house.) First, she looked in the (window) and saw that no one was (home.) So (Goldilocks) opened the (door) and went into the bears' (house.) There she saw the (bowls) of porridge on the (table.) There was a little (bowl) for the little (bear,) a middle-sized (bowl) for the middle-sized (bear,) and a big (bowl) for the big (bear.)

Example - Verbs

The parent or therapist must present the child with a paragraph something like the one below and have the child find all the verbs in the paragraph.

After the bears (made) porridge for breakfast, they (poured) it in the bowls to (cool) and (went) for a walk. Then a little Girl named Goldilocks (came) to the bears' house. First, she (looked) in the window and (saw) that no one (was) home. So Goldilocks (opened) the door and (went) into the bears' house. There she (saw) the bowls of porridge on the table. There (was) a little bowl for the little bear, a middle-sized bowl for the middle-sized bear, and a big bowl for the

Example - Pronouns

The parent or therapist must present the child with a paragraph something like the one below and have the child find all the pronouns in the paragraph.

After the bears made porridge for breakfast, they poured it in the bowls to cool and went for a walk. Then a little girl named Goldilocks came to the bears' house. First, she looked in the window and saw that no one was home. So Goldilocks opened the door and went into the bears' house. There she saw the bowls of porridge on the table. There was a little bowl for the little bear, a middle-sized bowl for the middle-sized bear, and a big bowl for the big bear.

Example - Prepositions

The parent or therapist must present the child with a paragraph something like the one below and have the child find all the prepositions in the paragraph.

(After) the bears made porridge for breakfast, they poured it (in) the bowls to cool and went for a walk. Then a little girl named Goldilocks came (to) the bears' house. First, she looked (in) the window and saw that no one was home. So Goldilocks opened the door and went (into) the bears' house. There she saw the bowls of porridge (on) the table. There was a little bowl (for) the little bear, a middle-sized bowl (for) the middle-sized bear, and a big bowl (for) the big bear.

Example - Adjectives

The parent or therapist must present the child with a paragraph something like the one below and have the child find all the adjectives in the paragraph.

After the bears made porridge for breakfast, they poured it in the bowls to cool and went for a walk. Then a little girl named Goldilocks came to the bears' house. First, she looked in the window and saw that no one was home. So Goldilocks opened the door and went into the bears' house. There she saw the bowls of porridge on the table. There was a little bowl for the little bear, a middle-sized bowl for the middle-sized bear, and a big bowl for the big bear.

5 Advanced Language Development

Story Writing
- Exercises

Story Pre-Writing
- Exercises

Topic Sentences
- Exercises

Paragraph Writing and Topical Conversation
- Exercises, and Scripts

Finding the Main Idea
- Scripts, and Exercises

Letter Writing
- Exercises

Recall of Significant Daily Events
- Exercises

Teaching Advanced Language Skills

Chapter 5, Advanced Language Development, concentrates on the language skills children need throughout their school years. The first section teaches story writing at a variety of levels, beginning with the most basic. By second grade, normally developing children are required to write simple stories at school. Some children with pervasive developmental disorders can keep up with their peers as long as they have been taught a structure they can use.

Once the child has a basic understanding of the structure of a story, we introduce story pre-writing. Story pre-writing is a way the child can prepare to write a story that is more complex in structure. The story pre-writing section provides exercises to teach the child how to set up a story and make an outline. Story pre-writing is a valuable tool for these children since as their normally developing peers become better readers and spellers, the teachers expectations of the class increase dramatically. Story pre-writing gives the bright language-delayed child an important way to keep up with the class.

The next section in the Advanced Language skills chapter goes into more depth with the written word by teaching the child how to identify a topic sentence and write a paragraph. This is a particularly important skill since reading <u>comprehension</u> is a weakness in most children with autism. By teaching the child to discern the topic sentence, s/he will have a much easier time understanding the paragraph.

The paragraph writing section further works on the child's ability to express him/herself with the written word in a way that is structured and follows the conventions of paragraph writing. Some normally developing children do not learn this skill until high school (or even college); however, for children with language delays, this structure is an important benefit and should be taught as soon as the child has completed all the story writing and pre-writing exercises.

The Finding the Main Idea section presents another exercise designed to work on the child's reading comprehension ability in nonfiction-like or descriptive paragraphs. The section teaches the child to create main ideas. Another exercise in this section has the child identify the main idea of nonfiction paragraphs. A structured technique by which the child learns to take notes from the descriptive paragraph is also introduced.

Letter writing is another skill children must learn since on many occasions they will need to write a letter to someone they know. Once the child learns to letter write, then thank you notes and holiday cards will become an easy task. Letter writing also gives the child an opportunity to communicate with someone through the written word which is often much easier than oral communication for children with language disorders.

The Recall of Significant Daily Events section works on a skill that is extremely difficult for most language delayed children. In this section, the child is taught to recall (from memory) what happened in his/her day. This skill takes years for some children to acquire; however, it is worth pursuing because it builds many other important skills as well. An additional benefit is some knowledge of what is happening in the child's day when the parent is not there to observe.

Note: All the exercises in this chapter use work sheets to visually prompt the child. Although it is tempting to allow the child to use the work sheet on a permanent basis, it is VERY important to fade the work sheet when the child has a firm grasp of the exercise. Otherwise, the child will continue to require work sheets to complete any assignment. Reliance on work sheets does not foster true independence. For some of the exercises a visual prompt will always be necessary; therefore, the child should become accustomed to working with lined paper used in the school system to create his/her outlines. This should be done ONLY when the child is very comfortable with the skill.

How To Teach Story Writing

Easy

The easy story template is provided on the next page. Initially, the therapist should select the subject/title of the story. It should include an agent (boy, girl, animal, etc...) and either a place, (e.g. at the zoo, at the park) or an action (e.g. eating lunch, playing with friends). The therapist should write the title on the title line. The first story line is self explanatory. For the second story line, the therapist may have to supply HIS or HER before name, and then have the child come up with a name (note: this may be hard for the child, so the therapist should give the child choices). For the next line, the child should say: "One day, (name) went or was ...," followed by whatever is in the title (e.g. to the park). It is important to always put the story into the past tense since it is easier to use the past tense than the different variations of present tense. This exercise is designed to work on story telling and not verb tenses. For work on verb tenses, see Chapter 6 - Using The Correct Verb Tense.

For the last three lines, the therapist must supply the verbs for each sentence following, First, Next, Last. (e.g. First, she saw...). The child must then finish the sentence for each line.

After the child generates the story, the therapist should have him/her read it aloud, and ask simple comprehension questions: "Where did the girl/boy go?"; "What was the boy's/ girl's name?" etc. Eventually, the therapist should take the form away, and have the child retell the story and answer the questions again. When retelling the story, it does not have to be word for word, but sequence is important. The actions first, next, and last need to be retold in that order since the main idea behind the story writing drill is logical sequencing. Gradually, the child will be required to add most of the story elements as the therapist provides less prompts. It is important for the child to understand how to put a simple story together first. It is a good idea to save the stories to see progress and to make sure the child is not recycling the same story to different people working with him/ her. Once the child has internalized the structure, s/he should be required after every story to retell the story without the form.

Note: There is no cause for worry if the sentences do not come easily at first. Any suggestion the child gives should be accepted as long as it is relevant to the activity or setting on the subject/title line.

Why Introduce Story Writing?

The purpose of this drill is to get the child to be able to create a logically sequenced story, to develop reading comprehension, and to facilitate his/her imagination. All these skills are required throughout the child's school years starting in first or second grade. Giving the child a structure for story-writing will greatly help him/her meet the language arts challenges s/he will encounter.

Easy Story Writing

Below is a sample of the easiest story template. It should be completed by the therapist with the child helping until the child understands the structure. The child should work on the easy story template until s/he can complete it, with no prompts whatsoever. Eventually, the child should be able to tell a story orally without using the sheet.

Easy Story Writing

(Subject/Title) _____A Girl at the Park._____

Once upon a time there was a _____girl_____ .

Her_____ name was _Sue._____

One day _Sue went to the park._____

First, _she went down the slide._____

Next, _she ran to the swings._____

Last, _she saw a dog._____

How To Teach Story Writing

Intermediate

This story writing form must be used with an EASY STORY PRE-WRITING FORM (in the next section of Chapter 5). Using the same structured story form provided, the therapist should let the child create the story on his/her own as in the initial story making activity. The therapist may have to prompt the child to make the pronoun agree with the noun. For example, if the story is about a girl, then HER name was Jane. After each main statement, the child should be prompted to elaborate on the original statement. For example, if the child says: "First she played games.", an elaboration would be, "She played Candyland". For the statement, "Next she ate ice-cream" an elaborative sentence would be, "It was chocolate". The elaborate statements must be prompted initially by the therapist saying, for example, "Tell me something about the ice cream". (prompt) "It was ".........". After the child generates the story, the therapist should 1) have him/her read it aloud and 2) ask the child simple comprehension questions as before. Then, the form should be taken away, and the child should retell the story and answer questions again. This may be difficult for the child to do at first because the story will be longer. Initially, the story should be written using one character. Once the child knows how to write a story about one girl/boy/man/woman, then the story can be written about two children/boys/girls/people (e.g. for the title "Two Girls At The Zoo").

Difficult

This story writing form must be used with an DIFFICULT STORY PRE-WRITING FORM (in the next section of this chapter). As the child progresses, the therapist can continue to expand on this structure. Eventually the child should be able to write paragraphs with one main idea and many sentences explaining and elaborating on that main idea (which is the correct way to structure a paragraph for all writers). In addition, the child should be taught to create stories where the characters speak to one another. At this stage of writing, the child is taught to describe the characters in detail.

Advanced

This story writing form must be used with an ADVANCED STORY PRE-WRITING FORM (in the next section of this chapter). At this stage of writing, the child is taught to outline the actual sequence of events that will create the story. A number of related paragraphs which include main ideas and details make up a long piece of prose. By increasing the number of related paragraphs and slightly modifying the pre-writing sheet (introduced shortly), the story writing structure can be modified to meet the needs of older students.

Why Teach Advanced Story-Writing?

The ability of an adult with a developmental disorder to express him/herself through writing will often determine the degree to which complex communication is possible for that person. Not only is this skill going to help throughout his/her school years, it will also give that person freedom to communicate with others. Since oral communication is so difficult, it is a major strength if people with language disorders can coherently express their thoughts on paper.

Intermediate Story Writing

This is a sample of the intermediate story template. It should be introduced once the child understands the structure of the easy template. The intermediate template introduces the idea of elaborative descriptive sentences (using another sentence to elaborate on the original sentence in a descriptive way). The child should work on this template until it is easy to complete independently.

Intermediate Story Writing

(Subject/Title) __A Girl at the Zoo__

Once upon a time there was __a girl.__

Her __name __was Jane.__

One day __Jane went to the zoo.__
  __The zoo was big.__

First, __she saw the monkeys.__
  __The monkeys were swinging.__

Next, __she went to the giraffes.__
  __The giraffes had long necks.__

Last, __she ate an ice-cream cone.__
  __The ice-cream cone was cold.__

Difficult Story Writing

This is a sample of the difficult story template. It should be introduced once the child understands the structure of the intermediate template. The difficult template introduces the idea of conversation within a story and emphasizes its structure.

Difficult Story Writing

(Subject/Title) _____Two Boys at Disneyland_____

Once upon a time there were two boys. Their names were Dave and Mike. One day, Dave and Mike went to Disneyland.

First,____Dave____ and _____Mike_____ rode on the roller coaster. Mike said, "That was fun". Dave said, "Yeah. Let's go to the Haunted Mansion.

After____ riding the roller coaster,____ Dave____ and ___Mike ran to the Haunted Mansion. Dave said, "Let's wait in line". Mike said, "o.k. "

Last _Mike_ and ___Dave___ went to buy some food. Mike said, "I want to eat a hamburger." Dave said, "I want to eat a hot dog". The boys went to the restaurant.

Advanced Story Writing

This is a sample of the advanced story template. It should be introduced once the child understands the structure of the difficult template. This template introduces the idea of character development within a story and builds upon the structure of the difficult story template. As the child becomes better at story writing, it is important to introduce other ways to start a story besides "Once upon a time" (e.g. One day...).

Advanced Story Writing

(Subject/Title) Two Boys Who Get Lost At Disneyland

Once upon a time there were two boys. Their names were Dave and Mike. Dave was 9 years old and short. He loved to eat fruit. John was 15 years old and big. He liked to eat marshmallows. One day, Dave and Mike went to Disneyland.

First, Dave and Mike got lost. Dave said, "Where's Mom?" Mike said, "I can't see her. Maybe she's at the roller-coaster."

After getting lost, Dave and Mike ran to the roller coaster. Dave said, "Maybe she's at the Haunted Mansion." Mike said, "Let's look there." Mom wasn't there.

Last Mike and Dave looked at the burger place. They found Mom. Mike said, "I want to eat a hamburger." Dave said, "I want to eat a hot dog." The boys ordered the food.

How To Teach Story Pre-Writing

Easy

After the child is able to write stories using the easiest template provided, it is time to introduce the story pre-writing sheets. Story pre-writing is introduced as follows:

1. The therapist writes the title of the story e.g. <u>Two Girls at the Park</u> at the top of the story pre-writing form.

2. Next, the therapist has the child give the "Girls" or characters names, using the story pre-writing sheet.

3. Then, the therapist asks the child to tell her the setting, according to the title, which in this case is "The Park". At first, this will probably need to be entirely prompted; however, after the child understands the structure, s/he should be able to do this without prompting.

4. Then the therapist asks when the story takes place. Any time of day or season the child offers is fine (for example, in summer, at 2:00 o'clock, in the morning, or at lunch). This will likely need to be prompted at first.

Once the child has completed the story pre-writing form, then s/he should be helped to weave this information into the story, in the introductory paragraph. The child should be dictating the introductory paragraph to the therapist who should write the story on the intermediate story-writing form. So, for example, the first paragraph should go something like this: "Once upon a time there was a girl. Her name was Sue. One day she went to the park. It was in the afternoon."

Difficult

The more difficult pre-writing form is used in much the same way as the easy form except that the child must give more information about the characters. The child must name two characters, describe the characters, describe the setting and give the time. Then the child must weave the information into the story after the first sentence which states that the story is about two children. For example, "Their names were Susan and Tony. Susan was 8 years old and had brown hair. Tony was 9 years old and had black hair. One day Susan and Tony went to the park". In this example, the child gives the two characters names, ages, and hair color. It is important that the descriptions of the characters vary; otherwise, the child will always use the same words to describe the characters. In addition, the setting and time must be discussed in more detail e.g. "Park, swings, slide, grass", and "2:30 in the afternoon".

Advanced

Once the child has mastered the easy and difficult pre-writing sheets, then the therapist should introduce the next stage which outlines the sequence of events paragraph by paragraph. All the information in the pre-writing sheet needs to be incorporated into the story.

Why Use A Pre-Writing Sheet?

The pre-writing sheet gives the child a structure to follow in order to be able to describe the various details that occur in a story. Not only does the pre-writing sheet help the child create a better story, it also helps the child comprehend stories that others have written since the child recognizes the implicit structure of the story. In addition, the pre-writing exercise helps the child differentiate between important parts of a story and the more descriptive, less important details that can make a story more colorful or interesting.

Easy Story Pre-Writing

This is a sample of the easy pre-writing template. It should be introduced once the child understands the structure of the easiest story template. Story Pre-Writing teaches the child to make an outline of the story that s/he will write. In this easy form, the outline has the child come up with the names of the characters, the setting and when the story takes place. This pre-writing sheet is for a story titled "Two Girls at the Park".

Easy Story Pre-Writing

Subject/Title: _Two Girls At The Park_

Characters: _Kate and Sue_

Setting: _park_

Time: _in the afternoon_

Difficult Story Pre-Writing

This is a sample of the Difficult Pre-writing template. It should be introduced once the child understands the structure of the easiest pre-writing template. In this form, the outline has the child describe his/her characters, elaborate on the setting and give a more in-depth idea of when the story takes place. *Note: Either the therapist gives the topic, or the child chooses a topic. If the child chooses, it is important that the child suggests a different topic each time the exercise is done.*

Difficult Story Pre-Writing

Story Title: Two Girls At The Park

Characters: Kate   and   Sue

(how old)	10 years old	5 years old
(what they like)	liked pizza	liked hamburgers
(a descriptive e.g. big, tall, small)	played the piano	good swimmer

Setting: Park

sand,

swings

slide

Time: Summer,

in the afternoon,

Tuesday,

3:00

Advanced Story Pre-writing

This is a sample of the Advanced Pre-writing template. It should be introduced once the child understands the structure of the preceding pre-writing templates. This work sheet actually constitutes an entire outline of a story from a description of the characters, an elaboration on the setting, an idea of when the story takes place to the actual sequence of events. At this stage, the child should be filling out his/her own pre-writing form.

Advanced Story Pre-writing

Story Title: _Two Boys Who Get Lost At Disneyland_

Characters:

David	John
9 years old	15 years old
short	big
eats fruit	eats marshmallows

Setting: _Disneyland_
rides
scary roller coaster, ferris wheel

Time: _Sunday_

STORY and SEQUENCE:

Paragraph 1: from above

Paragraph 2: First _David_ and _John got lost._

Paragraph 3: After _getting lost_, _David_ and _John looked for Mom._

Paragraph 4: Last _David_ and _John found Mom._

How To Teach Topic Sentences

The first step to introducing the concept of topic sentence is to read aloud, with the child, the Topic Sentence Script which describes and defines topic sentences. Then the therapist should ask the child questions about topic sentences based on the six lines read. For example, the child should be asked, "What can a topic sentence describe?" Then the therapist should fill in the Writing a Topic Sentence sheet based upon the topic given by the child. The first few times this activity is done, the therapist should heavily prompt the child with the correct answer until s/he is able to come up with a reasonably good topic sentence (a sentence that is connected to the topic). The topic chosen should be very familiar to the child. At first, the topic can be identical to a topic which was introduced in chapter 3 on animals, professions, sports etc... After the child understands what a topic sentence is, then the topics given can be those which the child is not intimately familiar with but knows something about.

Once the child has completed this activity sheet, it is a good idea to help him/her write a paragraph based on the topic sentence that s/he has written. At first, this can be heavily prompted by asking the child, "What else can you say about ___(xxx)___ ". In time, writing a paragraph should become relatively easy for the child to do.

Another activity which brings across the concept of topic sentence has the child recognize the topic sentence in a paragraph. The child should be given a paragraph and instructed to circle or underline the topic sentence. It is important that the topic sentence of the paragraphs be in the first or second line of the paragraph so as not to confuse the child. Since most topic sentences do appear in the first two lines, looking at the first two sentences to find the topic sentence is a good strategy for the child to follow.

Note: It is important that the script is read every time the activity is done, until the therapist is sure that the child understands the concept.

Why Teach Topic Sentences?

Once the child has learned to write a basic story (using the very structured format introduced to him), s/he must be given the tools to adapt that structure to nonfiction or fact-based writing since this kind of writing will be required from the child throughout his/her schooling. Teaching the child about topic sentences gives him/her an anchor from which to write the paragraph. This skill can be expanded to eventually writing an entire essay or book report. The child simply must create a number of topic sentences that relate to each other (in other words, an outline) and then build a paragraph around each topic sentence. It makes good sense to teach the structure of writing early and explicitly to children with autism since they thrive on structure. This approach gives the language delayed or autistic child an advantage over his normally developing peers.

Writing a Topic Sentence

This script teaches the child how to write a topic sentence. The therapist should introduce the script by reading the script with the child and asking the child questions about topic sentences.

Writing a Topic Sentence

- A Topic sentence is a sentence that tells the main idea of a topic.

- You can write many different kinds of topic sentences.

- A topic sentence can describe a topic.

- A topic sentence can tell how you feel about a topic. It gives your opinion.

- A topic sentence can compare a topic with something else.

- A topic sentence can give information about a topic.

Writing a Topic Sentence Exercise

This exercise teaches the child to write a topic sentence. After the child has read the script about topic sentences (on the preceding page), the therapist gives a topic and the child writes two topic sentences. At first, the therapist will need to prompt the child to complete the exercise; however, once the child understands how to complete this exercise, s/he should complete it independently. Eventually, the therapist should remove the sheet altogether and ask the child to orally create a topic sentence.

Writing a Topic Sentence

For each topic below, write 2 different topic sentences.

Topic: _School_

Topic Sentence #1: _My school is a fun place._
Topic Sentence #2: _I do lots of things at school._

Topic: _The Mall_

Topic Sentence #1: _The mall is a big place._

Topic Sentence #2: _I buy stuff at the mall._

Topic: _The Zoo_

Topic Sentence #1: _The Zoo is my favorite place._
Topic Sentence #2: _Many animals live in the Zoo._

How To Teach Paragraph Writing and Topical Conversation

At this level, paragraph writing and topical conversation have a very similar structure and can therefore be taught using the same instruments. The major difference is that in paragraph writing, the conversation is written down, whereas in topical conversation, the child orally gives the same information.

The activities are presented at three levels. At the first level (easy), the therapist asks the child what s/he would like to talk about. When the child gives the topic, the therapist should write the topic on the sheet. Then the therapist asks the child what s/he wants to say about the topic. The child may need some help to give a main idea as opposed to a detail. Once the child understands the difference between a main idea and a detail, s/he should be able to give a main idea independently. Then the child is asked to give four details (ideas) about the topic. The therapist should write the item down using one key word only. Once the child has finished giving ideas, s/he should be asked to either write his/her ideas down in full sentences (if the skill being worked on is paragraph writing) or tell about the topic in full sentences orally (if conversation skills are being practiced). The therapist will have to prompt the child heavily at the beginning; however, once the child understands the drill, s/he should be able to do this independently.

Once the child can easily complete the first level of paragraph writing, the second level (intermediate) should be introduced. The therapist should prompt the child to say one more thing about each detail. When first introducing the concept of elaborative phrases, anything the child suggests that is related to the main detail should be accepted. Once the child can easily elaborate (using one word), then the therapist should prompt the child to elaborate in a way that compares the details. For example, the child should elaborate on what can be bought in each store rather than making statements about each store that are unrelated. As with the easy level, the therapist should have the child write out a paragraph or tell about a topic using full sentences, following the outline.

The third level (advanced) is much the same as the first two, except that each main detail has three elaborative phrases relating to it, rather than one. The therapist should introduce this third level in much the same way as the other two levels. At this level, the child should be encouraged to use the outline to discuss the material as well as to write paragraphs from the material. Once the child can talk about the topic, then the sheet should be faded and the child should be required to talk about the topic from memory. For written paragraphs, the sheet never needs to be faded since using an outline is a natural thing to do when writing a paragraph, story, or essay.

Why Use Outlines To Teach These Skills?

Outlines give children with auditory processing problems a visual prompt, thereby giving them the opportunity to work on their expressive weaknesses. The outline for writing paragraphs gives them a tool to organize their thoughts in a way that is standard practice, using the structure that is universally accepted across academic settings.

Outline for Paragraph Writing and Topical Conversation - Easy

This exercise teaches the child the structure of a paragraph (that a paragraph is about a topic and is made up of a main idea and details). This exercise gives the child a rigid structure with which to organize thoughts. Within this structure, the child will find it easier to be creative.

Outline for Paragraph Writing &Topical Conversation - Easy

TOPIC: _____ stores
(what you want to talk about)

MAIN IDEA: There are many kinds of stores
(what you want to say about the topic)

① Safeway

DETAILS:
(the important things you want to say about the main idea)

② Mervyn's

③ Home Hardware

④ Tower Records

Outline for Paragraph Writing and Topical Conversation - Intermediate

The intermediate level of this exercise teaches the child that within the structure of a paragraph there is room for elaboration. Although the rigid structure is still adhered to, each detail has an elaborative statement (which is typical in paragraphs).

Outline for Paragraph Writing and Topical Conversation - Intermediate

TOPIC:
(what you want to talk about)

stores

MAIN IDEA:
(what you want to say about the topic)

There are many kinds of stores

DETAILS:
(the important things you want to say about the main idea)

(1) Safeway
   food

(2) Mervyn's
   clothes

(3) Home Hardware
   tools

(4) Tower Records
   music

Outline for Paragraph Writing and Topical Conversation - Advanced

The advanced version of this exercise shows that an essay, report, or paper has a main paragraph which introduces the subject of the paragraphs in the body of the writing, and that each paragraph in the body has its own main idea and details. Elaborative statements can be introduced here as the next step.

Outline for Paragraph Writing and Topical Conversation - Advanced

TOPIC: _____ stores _____

MAIN IDEA(S): _____ place to buy things _____
_____ many different kinds _____
_____

Paragraph
Topic: (1) Safeway _____

              Details: _____ groceries _____
_____ medicine _____
_____ paper goods _____

Paragraph
Topic: (2) Mervyn's _____

              Details: _____ clothes _____
_____ shoes _____
_____ jewelry _____

Paragraph
Topic: (3) Tower Records

              Details: _____ music tapes _____
_____ CDs _____
_____ videos _____

Paragraph
Topic: (4) Orchard Supply

              Details: _____ tools _____
_____ paint _____
_____ plants _____

How To Teach Paragraph Writing

Advanced

Prerequisite: Before paragraph writing can be formally taught, the child should be quite good at story writing, story pre-writing and topic sentences (which are covered at the beginning of this chapter).

The first step in teaching paragraph writing is to introduce the script, "How To Write a Paragraph". This script should be read to and talked about with the child a few times before actually beginning to teach paragraph writing. The script should be presented either on a black board or on a large sheet of paper to make it easier for the child to follow along. The child should come to understand that a paragraph has three parts, one of which (topic sentences) the child knows how to create already.

Once the child understands the script to a reasonable degree, then the "Writing a Paragraph" sheet should be worked on with the therapist. The child should choose the topic (which should interest the child) and then create a main idea or topic sentence. At first, the child may need prompting to give details about the topic rather than giving another main idea. In addition, the concluding sentence may need to be prompted, at first. After a few times, the child should recognize the structure of a paragraph. If the child is not internalizing this structure, it is possible that s/he did not really understand the drills which preceded this activity i.e. topic sentences; therefore, in this situation it is a good idea to go back and spend more time on topic sentences.

Once paragraph writing seems easy for the child, it is time to move on to story development. The "Developing Your Story" sheets combine all the skills the child has been working on up to this point -- Story Writing, Story Pre-writing, Topic Sentences, and Paragraph Development. Story development is a very advanced skill which is important to teach when the child is ready, and not before. It is important to keep this in mind because premature introduction of this may create frustration which should be avoided whenever possible since it can derail an otherwise successful language program. Although story development can be difficult, it is an important skill to learn for the child to keep up with his/her peers in a mainstream setting.

Why Teach Paragraph Writing?

Paragraph writing is important to teach because it is a foundation skill that the child needs to participate fully in any mainstream academic curriculum. Fortunately, normally developing children do not develop these skills for many years. By making the structure explicit, developmentally delayed children are able to keep up in this area of language arts. In addition, some children eventually may find it easier to communicate complex thoughts using the written word. This gives them the tools necessary to express themselves in nonverbal ways.

How To Write a Paragraph

This is a script that should be read with the child many times and, through repetition and asking questions, taught to the child. Once the child begins to understand the structure of a paragraph, then the activity sheets that follow should be introduced.

All scripts should be introduced on a large sheet of paper, blackboard, or dry-erase board.

How To Write a Paragraph

A PARAGRAPH IS A GROUP OF SENTENCES THAT ARE ALL ABOUT ONE IDEA OR TOPIC.

You can write a paragraph about anything you want to.

EVERY PARAGRAPH NEEDS TO HAVE 3 MAIN PARTS.

The 3 main parts of a paragraph look like this:

1. **<u>A TOPIC SENTENCE</u> ---> this sentence tells exactly what the paragraph is about. It is the main idea sentence.**

   If you wanted to write about baseball, a topic sentence might be, *"Baseball is a team sport."*
   If you wanted to write about school, a topic sentence might be, *"You can learn many things at school".*

2. **<u>At least 3 SUPPORTING SENTENCES</u>---> these are detail sentences that "back up" your topic sentence.**

   If you were writing about school, 3 supporting sentences might be:
   Math is one of the things you learn to do at school.
   You also learn to read and spell at school.
   At school, you learn to write stories and paragraphs about many different things.

3. **<u>A CONCLUDING SENTENCE</u> ---> this is usually the last sentence in your paragraph. It is a summary of your topic. The concluding sentence retells the main idea.**

   If you were writing about school, your concluding sentence might be, *"Going to school teaches you many different things."*
   If you wanted to write about school, a topic sentence might be: *"You can learn many things at school".*

*REMEMBER: NO MATTER WHAT KIND OF PARAGRAPH YOU WRITE, IT NEEDS TO HAVE THE 3 MAIN PARTS.

Writing a Paragraph

This sheet is designed to make explicit the structure of a paragraph. It will make it easier for the child to write paragraphs and will hopefully improve the child's story writing as well.

Writing a Paragraph

TOPIC: _Discovery Zone_

Topic Sentence:
(main idea)

The Discovery Zone is a fun place to go.

3 Supporting Sentences:
(Details)

1. _They have balls, slides and tubes at the Discovery Zone._

2. _You can eat pizza, popcorn and ice-cream there._

3. _You can play games and win prizes at the Discovery Zone._

Concluding Sentence:
(Summary sentence that retells the main idea)

I like to go to the Discovery Zone.

Developing Your Story (Introductory Paragraph)

The following four sheets give the child the opportunity to put all the various parts of a story together in one outline. This sheet lays out the topic sentence in the first paragraph and joins it with character development and elaborative sentences. The following sheets help the child develop the paragraphs within the story.

Developing Your Story (Introductory Paragraph)

STORY TITLE: _Two Boys Who Get Lost At Great America_

INTRODUCTORY PARAGRAPH

Topic Sentence: _This is the story about two kids named David and John._

Supporting Details:
(Character Description)
David was 9 years old and very short.
He liked to eat fruit.

(Character Description)
John was 15 years old and very big.
He liked to eat marshmallows.

SETTING/TIME PARAGRAPH

Topic Sentence: _On Sunday, David and John went to Great America._

Supporting Details:
There were lots of rides.
There was a scary roller coaster.
There was a red and blue ferris wheel.

Developing Your Story - Paragraph 2

This sheet lays out the topic sentence in the second paragraph and joins it with detail sentences which support the topic sentence.

Developing Your Story - Paragraph 2

EVENT PARAGRAPH (1)

Topic Sentence: First, David and John got lost.

_____

Supporting Details (3 Sentences of Support):

1. They couldn't find Mom.

_____

_____

2. David said, "oh, no, we're lost."

_____

_____

3. John shouted, "Mom where are you?"

_____

_____

Developing Your Story - Paragraph 3

This sheet lays out the topic sentence in the third paragraph and joins it with detail sentences which support the topic sentence.

Developing Your Story - Paragraph 3

EVENT PARAGRAPH (2)

Topic Sentence: _____After getting lost, David and John looked for Mom._____

Supporting Details (3 Sentences of Support):

1. They looked for Mom on the roller coaster ride. Mom was not there.

2. They looked for Mom on the ferris wheel. Mom was not there.

3. They looked for Mom at the snack stand. Mom was not there.

Developing Your Story - Paragraph 4

This sheet lays out the topic sentence in the fourth and concluding paragraph and joins it with detail sentences which support the topic sentence.

Developing Your Story - Paragraph 4

EVENT PARAGRAPH (3)

Topic Sentence: _Last, David and John found Mom._

Supporting Details (3 Sentences of Support):

1. _They found Mom on the log ride._

2. _They shouted, "Mom, there you are."_

3. _They were happy._

How To Teach Finding the Main Idea

Prerequisite: The child has already been introduced to simple paragraphs, such as those in the general information chapter.

The first step to teaching the concept of "Finding the Main Idea", is to read the script titled, "How To Find The Main Idea", on the following page. It should be read with the child several times so that the child becomes comfortable with the structure of the exercise. Once s/he understands the instructions, then an easy paragraph should be introduced. Samples of easy paragraphs follow.

When introducing the easy paragraph, the therapist should have the child read the entire paragraph first. Then, using the script, the therapist should ask the child, "What is the <u>one</u> subject the author is talking about in the paragraph?" . Once the child answers, then the therapist should ask, "What is the author saying about the topic?" Then the child should be asked to underline the topic sentence -- the sentence with the main idea in it. The child will come to understand that the main idea is usually (unfortunately not always) in the first and/or second line of the paragraph. Once the child has successfully underlined the topic sentence, then s/he should be instructed to find the details and circle them.

Once the child understands these simple descriptive paragraphs, slightly more difficult paragraphs should be introduced. The goal is for the child to <u>eventually</u> be able to read and comprehend quite advanced descriptive paragraphs such as those found in nonfiction, academic books.

Another exercise to improve this skill is "Finding the Main Idea" through the use of lists. The child should look at a list of words provided by the therapist and be prompted to identify the category from the examples. Once s/he can do that, then the child should be instructed to 1) write the category beside the "Main Idea" heading, 2) write the details next to the "Details" heading, and 3) create a topic sentence based on the list. This activity should be done many times with different lists so the child can identify the pattern.

The next drill, "Sentence Starters For Descriptive Topic Sentences and Detail Sentences of Support", works on the same skill but at a higher level. The therapist should have the child fill in the blanks with help until it becomes easy. In this way, the relationship between the main idea and details is further solidified and the child is given various structures to use when writing about both main ideas and details.

The "Two-Column Notes" form is for the child to use when taking notes from a paragraph. The child should write the various parts of the paragraph in the appropriate place on the form so that at a glance the child will be able to understand what the paragraph is about. This should be done in point form, not in whole sentences.

Why Teach Finding the Main Idea?

Teaching a child how to find the main idea is critical for the child's comprehension skills and ability to write clearly and express ideas to others. Without this skill, the child is unable to understand what information to concentrate upon and what to ignore.

How To Find The Main Idea

This script should accompany a paragraph for the child to work on. Examples of such paragraphs are on the next page. The child should do this with all descriptive paragraphs until these ideas are internalized. This will increase comprehension levels.

This script should be introduced to the child on a full size sheet of paper

How To Find The Main Idea

A. Read **EACH** paragraph and answer these questions:

- **Topic:** What is the one subject the author is talking about in the paragraph?

- **Main Idea**: What is the author saying about the topic?

- **Details:** What details support the main idea?

B. Find and underline the **TOPIC SENTENCE** that states this main idea.

C. Circle any **DETAILS** that support the topic sentence in each paragraph.

Descriptive Paragraphs

(1) People live in many different kinds of homes. Many people live in houses. A house is a home. Some people live in an apartment. The apartment is their home. Kings live in palaces. Palaces are very big homes with many rooms.

(2) You can learn many things at school. You can learn to do math at school. You learn addition, subtraction, multiplication, and division. Another thing you learn at school is how to read. You are taught to sound out words. You also learn to write and spell in school.

(3) Stores sell many different things. Some stores sell just groceries. Safeway is a grocery store. Other stores have clothes and jewelry for you to buy. Mervyn's sells lots of clothes. Computer stores sell computers, games, and other computer supplies.

Finding the Main Idea

This exercise is designed to work on the comprehension skills of the child without requiring the child to read a paragraph. This sheet can be introduced to the child before the outline for paragraph writing is introduced or once the child knows how to write a simple paragraph.

Finding the Main Idea

Look at each list. Determine the main idea and the details. Then write a topic sentence for your main idea.

List: doll   Main Idea: toys

wagon   *Details:* wagon

legos   legos

toys   doll

Topic Sentence: There are many different kinds of toys.

List: broccoli   Main Idea: vegetables

carrots   *Details:* carrots

vegetables   peas

peas   broccoli

Topic Sentence: There are many different vegetables

Sentence Starters For Descriptive Topic Sentences and Detail Sentences of Support

This exercise introduces the child to the structure of detail sentences and their relationship to topic sentences. The topic should be one which the child has learned about and knows well. This topic in the example corresponds to a paragraph in the general information chapter.

Sentence Starters For Descriptive Topic Sentences and Detail Sentences of Support

Topic Sentence: There are many kinds of _mammals_.

Detail Sentences:

A _n elephant_ is a kind of _mammal_.

One kind of _mammal_ is _an elephant_.

Another kind of _mammal_ is _a dolphin_.

A human being is also a kind of _mammal_.

Topic Sentence: A _mammal_ is a _n animal_ (that has/with/that can) _hair on its skin._

Detail Sentences:

For example, _an elephant_ is _a mammal_.

An example of _a mammal_ is _an elephant._

A _n elephant_ is an example of _a mammal_.

Another example of _a mammal_ is _a dolphin_.

A human being is also an example of _a mammal_.

Topic Sentence: _Mammals_ are _animals_ (that have/with/that can) _hair on their skin._

Detail Sentences:

One type of _mammal_ is _an elephant._.

A _n elephant_ is a type of _mammal_.

Another type of _mammal_ is _a dolphin._.

A human being is also a type of _a mammal._.

Two-Column Notes

This sheet is designed to help the child comprehend a descriptive paragraph by taking notes from that paragraph in a structured way. The sheet has room for three paragraphs that may be related to one another; however, when the child is learning this skill, each paragraph should be able to stand alone.
There are two columns so the child can glance at the left column and know what the paragraph is about without the details in the right column distracting him/her.

Two-Column Notes

What Is The Text About?

1st Paragraph	
Topic:	**Details:**
Tropical rain forests	hot and humid
	many different animals
Main Idea:	many insects
grow in central part	unusual plants
of earth	being cut down

2nd Paragraph	
Topic:	**Details:**
Tropical rain forest	gorilla, chimpanzees, orangutan, gibbon
apes	live in family groupings
Main Idea:	eat plants, insects and bird eggs.
apes are closest	live in treetops, or forest floor
relative to man	

3rd Paragraph	
Topic:	**Details:**
Tropical rain forests	tiger, ocelot, leopard, jaguar
cats	good eyesight, hearing, and smell
Main Idea:	active at night
several different kinds	camouflaged fir
live in rain forests	

How To Teach Letter Writing

The therapist should introduce letter writing by using a letter template that has the greeting, "Dear_(xxx)_, How are you?", and the ending, "Love, _(xxx)_". Once the therapist has written the greeting, she should prompt the child to create one sentence about any topic. For example, the child could say, "I like Power Rangers", or, "I went swimming". The therapist would then write, "Love", and prompt the child to sign his/her name. Then, during the next therapy session (the following day), the therapist does the same thing, but this time prompts the child to tell the therapist how to begin i.e. "Dear (xxx) ". As the letter drill is done repeatedly, the child memorizes the structure and the therapist can then prompt progressively less. Once the child has mastered this structure, then the therapist should have him/her say two things in the body of the letter. Eventually, the child will be able to write a letter by him/herself, telling about personal experiences and asking the recipient of the letter questions. This, however, will depend on the age of the child and must be done in steps, with the therapist gradually fading out old prompts and challenging the child with new, extended letter writing skills (such as asking questions).

Why Teach Letter Writing?

Letter writing is a skill that is easy for language-delayed children to learn because the basic structure of a letter does not vary considerably. In addition, the common opening of the letter and the closing of the letter take away the pressure of beginning and ending. This is also a good way for the child to practice communicating in a non-pressured format. In addition, if the child can correspond with a relative or friend, the questions asked by the correspondent will give the child an opportunity to answer questions.

Letter Template

This template introduces the child to letter writing. Letters can be quite structured which makes them fairly easy to master.

Letter Template

Date: June 20th, 1996

Greeting:

Dear Grandma,

Body: How are you? I'm good.

I went to Discovery Zone. It was

fun. I ate ice-cream and lots of

popcorn.

Closing: Love,

Name: Josh

How To Teach Recall of Significant Daily Events

Prerequisite: The child must understand the basic concept of before and after (which can be done through introducing sequence cards available from an educational supply store).

The therapist or parent should do this drill every day, right after the child returns from school. The adult asks, "What did you do today?" and the child must say one thing. The first few times, the child may have to be prompted. Once the child has mastered this, the adult should say, "Tell me three things you did today". The adult should cue the child by counting off on the adult's fingers. The child should be prompted to do this, since cuing often helps the child remember. This will be quite difficult for the child at first, and most of the answers will be by rote e.g. "I went to school, I ate lunch, I played on the swings". When the child can do this by rote, the adult should require a recall of 5 things. In order to stop the child from relying on the rote answers, it is a good idea to ask questions about particular subjects e.g.. "What did you do in math". "Did you have P.E. today?" "Who did you play with at recess?" Once the child answers the question, then the adult asks again, "Tell me 5 things you did in school today". The child should then be able to recall the subjects that the adult has asked the child about. **This is an important step and should not be omitted.** This drill should be done until the child has no problem recalling his/her day in a non-memorized, original manner. This may take some time -- possibly years -- but it is important since it teaches the child about sequencing (which will be discussed in more depth in Chapter 6).

There are several ways to make this drill easier for the child. One method is for the child's teacher or aide at school to help the child write down, on a small note pad, a few interesting things that happened to the child each day. Then, when the child is asked to recall his/her day, s/he can flip open the note pad and use each single word written about every activity to make a sentence. Eventually, the note pad can be faded out.

Another important thing to remember is that the information should be given in the correct order; therefore, when the adult prompts the child, the adult should say, "What did you do at school today?". "What happened FIRST?". The child should answer, "First, I _(xxx)_ ", Then I _(xxx)_ , and "Last I _(xxx)_ ". Eventually, the first, next, then, and last structure can be dropped; however, this structure should be used until the child internalizes the concept that the recall of activities need to be in their correct sequence.

Another way to make this drill easier is to use the "What Did You Do Today" activity sheet provided opposite. The therapist should ask who the child played with, what s/he saw, what s/he ate, etc. The topic should be put in the large center circle and the child's answers should be written in the small circles.

Another way to bring across the idea of daily recall is to write the sequence of the child's day on a calendar -- EVERY DAY. This gives the child a visual representation of his/her day which gives the child a clearer understanding of what the adult wants to know.

NOTE: It is generally easier for a child to recall his day on the Weekend, since the school schedule is the same, day after day, which makes it difficult to find something of interest to talk about. On the weekend, though, the activities are often different.

Why Teach Routines of Daily Life?

Routines of Daily Life are a relevant way to teach children with delays about sequencing and time, which are crucial to their advanced language development. In addition, because these routines are highly relevant to the child, they are good topics to use to increase spontaneous language.

What Did You Do Today?

This form is to be used to help the child recall his/her day. Once the child remembers something, then it is written in one of the balloons. When all the spaces are full, the child uses this sheet to describe his/her day in full sentences. Then the sheet should be removed, and the child should recall that day orally (without the visual prompt). When the child can easily recall his/her day using the sheet, the sheet should not be used at all, and the child should be required to recall his day independently and orally. The eventual elimination of the sheet is very important.

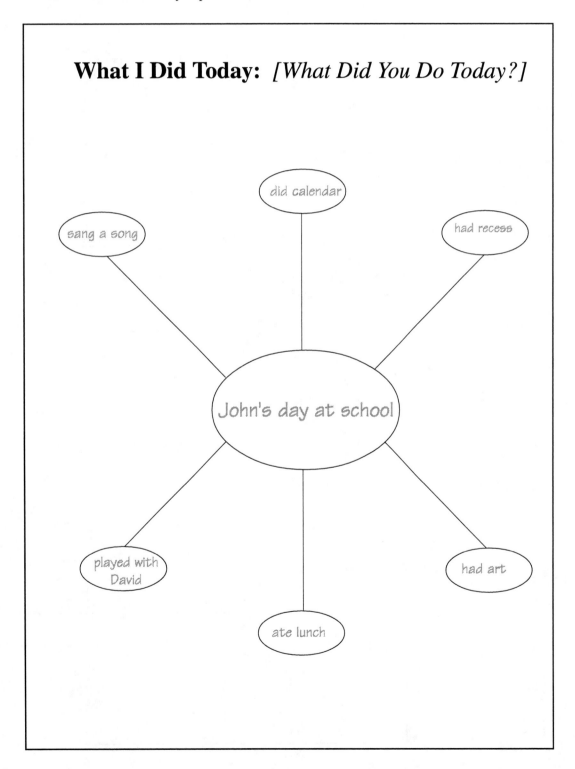

Daily Routine Sheet

This sheet is a written record of the child's recall of his/her day. The therapist or parent must write the child's recall word for word to be able to accurately gauge progress in recall from week to week. Note that this is NOT a sheet that the child works with directly.

Recall of Day

I went to summer camp.

I went swimming.

I ate lunch. I ate crackers.

I put on my bathing suit.

I played with Elena.

I went with Margaret.

I played tag.

6 Academics/Language Based Concepts

Categorization
- Exercises

Brainstorming
- Exercises

Pre-Reading Comprehension
- Exercises

Reading Comprehension
- Exercises

Math Word Problems
- Exercises

Vocabulary
- Exercises

Sequencing Concepts
- Numbers - Scripts and Exercises
- Money - Scripts and Exercises
- Time - Scripts and Exercises
- Daily Activities - Scripts and Exercises
- Calendar - Scripts and Exercises

Note-Taking
- Exercises

Agents and Their Actions
- Exercises

Verbal Analogies
- Exercises

Teaching New Concepts
- Exercises

A Chapter On Academics

Children with pervasive developmental disorders often excel in academic subjects. However, problems often arise by the way the subject matter is introduced and conveyed. This is the reason we emphasize academics. This chapter includes activities and drills designed to combat typical areas of weakness which confront children with autism spectrum disorders.

Lower Level Activities

The therapist should first introduce the following drills to the child: categorization (noun, verb, and simple categorization); familiar words: identifying group and function; object functions; brainstorming; and simple pre-reading comprehension (who, and did what). Although these drills do not seem to correspond directly to what is taught at school, these skills are the underpinnings of much academic skill.

Higher Level Activities

Throughout the child's school experience there will be several skills that require work. It is wise to begin working on these skills once the child has mastered the lower level skills and can decode relatively well (at a first grade level). These drills include: reading comprehension; math problems; vocabulary; sequencing; money; time; calendar; note-taking; agents and their actions.

1. Reading Comprehension

Comprehension is one of the most important deficits of children with pervasive developmental disorders. Therefore, it is important to start using the sheets included in this book as soon as the child can decode well. In addition, a reading comprehension series, such as Reading Milestones, should be started. Read the comprehension section in this chapter for more information.

2. Math Word Problems

Despite the child's ability at math, understanding and correctly completing math word problems is a major challenge for most children with language disorders. By following the math word problem drill set out in this book, the child becomes intimately familiar with math problems and is better able to solve math problems because s/he understands the pattern and purpose of the math word problem. This drill is NOT designed to teach math concepts. The purpose is to improve the child's understanding of the language involved in a math word problem.

3. Vocabulary

Children with language disorders do not typically learn new vocabulary from their normal environment. Therefore, it is important to teach new vocabulary in a way that the child does not just memorize the new vocabulary, but also uses that vocabulary. The vocabulary section in the book should be used once the child already has one word for every common object. To illustrate, a child who does not know the word for "dirt" should not be introduced to the word "soil". First the word "dirt" should be taught. A dictionary can be an invaluable tool for a child who has difficulty processing auditory information since a dictionary contains all the "answers" i.e. word definitions. It is important that a SIMPLE children's dictionary is used. The dictionary must be on the same level as is the child's decoding ability.

4. Number Sequencing
Since sequencing is often a major deficit for children with autism spectrum disorders, and a prerequisite to so many skills, sequencing is a skill that must be developed. The number sequencing is the simplest type of sequencing and should, therefore, be introduced first.

5. Money
Once number sequencing is mastered, then money can be introduced. The therapist should expect to work with the child on money for many months, if not years. It is a good idea to introduce money when the child's peers are taught it in school. It must be taught until the child understands money in its complexity (which usually is long after it is taught in school).

6. Time
Time is another of those skills that requires a good knowledge of sequencing. Time and Money can be taught concurrently; however, it is important to introduce one of them first and have the child work on the first concept for a month or so before introducing the second concept.

7. Calendar
Calendar should be introduced early on in a limited manner and practiced until the child understands the concept. This skill may also take a long time to master.

8. Note-Taking
Note-taking drills should be introduced once the child can print relatively quickly. A precocious first grader may be able to begin this drill, but typically the therapist should introduce this drill to a child once s/he can print, and receive and decode basic information through listening. This is a skill that is VERY IMPORTANT since the child who has difficulty focusing and understanding auditory instructions may be much more successful if s/he learns how to take notes on what is said without having to understand what is said at the same time. The child can then look at the notes which should give him/her a clue as to what is required. The teacher who writes instructions on the chalkboard is ideal for the child with a language-disorder; however, throughout school the child is not guaranteed to encounter this kind of teacher. Note-taking skills are taught to encourage independence. Therefore, this is also a skill that is important for a child who is not in a regular education class.

9. Agents and Their Actions, and Verbal Analogies
These two additional drills target two weaknesses in language which are often the foundation of a variety of academic skills. When the child masters these skills, s/he also improves academic critical thinking skills.

How To Teach Categorization

Prerequisite: The child should have been introduced to the concepts of categories using icons, cards or 3-dimensional materials before doing this drill.

This is one of the first drills that a child should learn to do. Using the form provided, the therapist should say:
Therapist: "Name something (in a specific group") or
        "Read the words. What group is this?"
If necessary, the therapist may need to read the words again and say,
Therapist: " banana, apple, orange. These are all things that are fruit."
After the child has generated 4 items or named the category, the therapist should have him/her verbalize what is written using complete sentences (e.g. "These are things that are round. A penny is round. The sun is round. A ball is round. A plate is round."). Initially, this drill will need to be modelled. Eventually, the child will be required to make an elaborative statement on each item that she names. For example, the child could say, "A ball is round. I bounce a ball."   The therapist should only write one or two words which represent what the child actually says. The one word acts as a cue to visually prompt the child to give a complete sentence.

Verbalization of what is written is as important as the actual generation of categorical items. This drill helps the child use complete sentences and maintain a verbalization for 4-5 sentences. As the child understands this activity better, the therapist can have the child talk about ,and eventually, write a paragraph about familiar categories e.g. "Suzie, tell me about things that are shiny." By the time the child is able to write well, the goal is for him/her to be able to write a coherent paragraph using this procedure. This drill works very well with some children.

At first, the drill should be done visually. Once the child understands the structure of the drill, the drill should be done visually and then verbally (without the visual prompt).
NOTE: The example used in the above paragraph is quite advanced. Examples of lower level categories are: things you eat; things you wear; things you ride; things you play with.

Why Teach Categorization?

The purpose of the categorization drill is 1) to develop the child's categorization skills, and 2) to enable him/her to verbalize how and/or why a group of words are related. Ability to categorize helps the child make more sense out of his/her world because categorization brings structure to the child's world.

Simple Categorization: Nouns

This activity is designed to teach the child simple noun categorization. When the child can complete this exercise with ease, the next drill should be introduced. The therapist should use this drill to probe for the level of the child. If the child cannot complete this drill, then s/he should be introduced to the concepts of categories using icons, cards or 3-dimensional materials (these precursor drills must precede use of the exercises in this book).

Simple Categorization: Nouns)

Name 4 items in each group.

1. <u>food</u>   (cake) (corn) (apple) (chips)

2. <u>animals</u>   (cow) (pig) (dog) (duck)

3. <u>toys</u>   (doll) (blocks) (lego) (crayon)

4. <u>vehicles</u>   (car) (boat) (train) (plane)

5. <u>clothes</u>   (shoes) (shirt) (pants) (dress)

Simple Categorization: Verbs

This activity is designed to teach the child simple verb categorization. If the child can do this drill easily, the next exercise should be introduced. If the child does not understand the concept of category, then s/he needs to be introduced to categories using icons, cards or 3-dimensional materials before being introduced to the exercises in this book.

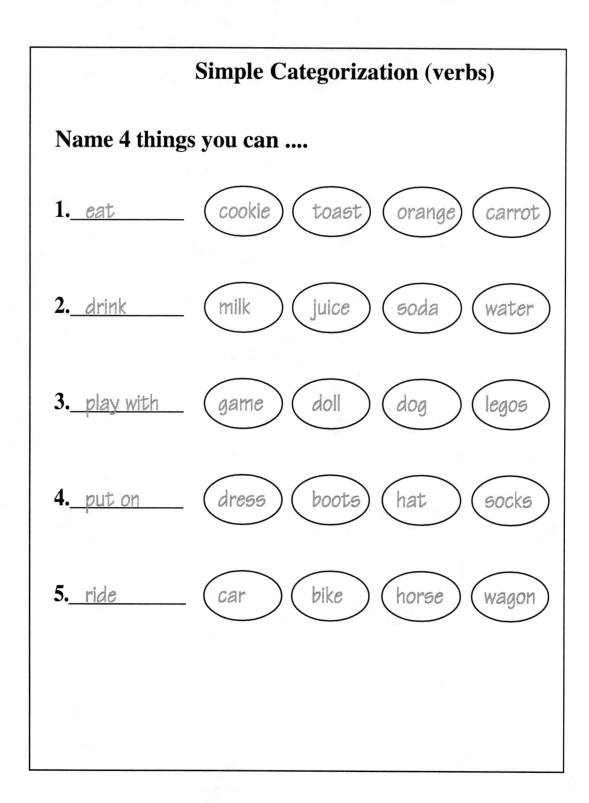

Simple Categorization (verbs)

Name 4 things you can ....

1. _eat_   cookie   toast   orange   carrot

2. _drink_   milk   juice   soda   water

3. _play with_   game   doll   dog   legos

4. _put on_   dress   boots   hat   socks

5. _ride_   car   bike   horse   wagon

Simple Categorization: Naming Items

This activity is a variation on the noun and verb categorization exercises. The focus in this drill is on the child's ability to name items that are in a category. The child should be able to complete the noun and verb categorization before being introduced to the Naming Items categorization exercise.

Simple Categorization: Naming Items

Write down four items that belong in each group.

food	animal	furniture
hotdog	monkey	chair
popcorn	lion	bed
hamburger	horse	sofa
ice-cream	elephant	table

Familiar Words: Identifying the Group & Function

This exercise is designed to teach the child the relationship between the object, the category (group) it is part of, and what it does (its function). This exercise should be introduced once the child has internalized several noun and verb categories.

Familiar Words: Identifying the Group and Function

Object	Group	Function
1. ball	toy	play with
2. pants	clothes	wear
3. chair	furniture	sit
4. shoe	clothes	put on
5. apple	fruit	eat

Object Functions: Fill-Ins

This exercise is designed to teach the child the relationship between the verb (action word) and the noun. This activity requires the child to find a verb which goes with the object. If the child can write, s/he can complete the sheet independently once s/he understands the structure of the drill.

Object Functions: Fill-Ins

Complete Each Sentence.

1. I _put on_ shoes.

2. I _eat_ pizza.

3. I _drink_ juice.

4. I _throw_ a ball.

5. I _sit in_ a chair.

Categorization

This exercise teaches the child to categorize activities that occur during a period of time. The child should be able to complete the noun and verb sheets with ease before this sheet is introduced. It is important that the child retell the therapist about the topic in complete sentences, first using the sheet as a visual prompt, and then without the sheet.

Things that are (or things I do at):

recess

1. climb

2. upside down

3. swing

4. jump rope

5. slide

6. run

How To Teach Brainstorming

The therapist writes a topic on the top of the Brainstorming form and has the child answer the following: "Tell me things that are _____", or "Tell me about things we do when _____." Once the child understands the drill, then the therapist can use less concrete categories. Note that the categories should be relevant to the child. For example, with two children the topic could be, "Things to do at Disneyland" or "Videos I like to watch." The more relevant the topic to the child, the more the child will be motivated to do the drill. Once the key word(s) is written down, then the therapist should go through the whole sheet and prompt the child to state each idea in a full sentence. This is a good drill to do with a typically developing peer in order to see what the peer's sentence structure looks like. It is important to remember that the child should be taught to speak like his/her peers and not like a robot or English professor. Once the child has created sentences using the key word, the sheet should be taken away and the child should be required to orally tell the therapist about the topic.

Why Teach Brainstorming?

Brainstorming helps the child answer a question or generate ideas on a topic without having to form a full sentence. The child's one word suggestions are then turned into sentences, which gives the child some ownership over the thought process. This also gives the therapist material to help the child improve his/her sentence structure. In addition, brainstorming shows the therapist what the child knows and what the child does not know (and therefore, needs to work on). Because this drill can be done with a typically developing peer, it gives the child a chance to interact verbally with a peer and learn to take turns.

Brainstorming

This exercise teaches the child to generate ideas without being constrained by the difficulty of putting the ideas into a sentence. Once the ideas have been generated, then the child can use the key words to talk about the subject in full sentences.

Brainstorming

Topic: _____Weather_____

○ rain _____   ○ _____wet_____

○ sunny _____   ○ _____cold_____

○ cloudy _____   ○ _____hot_____

○ foggy _____   ○ _____overcast_____

○ snowy _____   ○ _____warm_____

○ _____   ○ _____

How To Teach Pre-Reading Comprehension

It is recommended that the reader look at the example of the Pre-Reading Comprehension sheet while reading the "How To" section.

Prerequisite: Before starting the Pre-Reading Comprehension sheet, the therapist should go through the WHO list with the child saying, "the boy is a who. The man is a who" etc., emphasizing the words boy and who. The therapist should also introduce the "Did What" sheet using the DID WHAT list. The child should also read the lists in the same way as the therapist. Only then should the pre-reading comprehension sheet be introduced.

When introducing the pre-reading comprehension, the therapist must begin with a sheet that only contains <u>either</u> "Who?" or "Did What?" questions. The therapist should have the child read the short sentence. The therapist should repeat that short sentence so that the child can also hear the sentence read smoothly. The first few times the therapist should emphasize the part of the sentence that is going to relate to the question i.e. "THE BOY walked". Then when she asks "WHO walked?" the child will hear the similar inflection for the answer. Once the child understands the sentence and question, and can answer the question by circling the part of the sentence with the relevant word, then the therapist should stop using her voice as a prompt and ask the question in a normal, neutral tone. Once the child can answer simple "Who" questions" then it is time to introduce "What did?" questions in the same manner (using inflection at first until the child understands the relationship between "What Did?" and the action word). When the child can answer "What Did?" questions easily, then "Who" and "What Did" questions can be mixed in a random order (as is shown on the second Pre-Reading Comprehension sheet).

When the child is successful at this simple reading comprehension then the next reading comprehension exercises can be introduced.

Why Do Simple Comprehension Drills?

Some children with pervasive developmental disorders are great decoders; however, they general have great difficulty in comprehending what they are reading. Part of the difficulty may be due to the inability to sequence well. This difficulty may also be a result of having a limited vocabulary. These pre-comprehension drills are designed to make the child focus on two very important parts of the sentence, the person or "Who", and the action or "What did". Once the child learns to find and understand this important information in every sentence, s/he will be ready to begin story comprehension (which is introduced after these drills).

Who List

The "Who?" list is designed to precede the beginning comprehension drills. The therapist is to go over this list until the child understands that WHO is a person.

Who List

Who? =

the boy	**the girl**
the man	**the woman**
mom	**dad**
the baby	**the kids**
Michael	**Sue**
Mary	**Steven**

Did What List

The "Did What?" list is designed to precede the beginning comprehension drills. The therapist is to go over this list until the child understands that DID WHAT relates to an action (verb).

Did What List

Did What? =

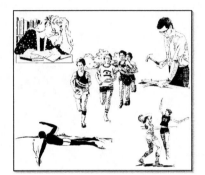

ate	jumped
cried	walked
played	slept
ran	swam
talked	read
stopped	clapped

Pre-Reading Comprehension: Who? and What did (or do)?

The child should read the sentence and then answer the question by circling the correct word in the sentence. This exercise should be introduced using only "Who" questions. Once the child can complete the sheet easily answering the "Who" questions without help, the same sheet should be used asking only "What Did _____ do?" questions. Once the child can answer these questions without prompts, then the "Who" and the "What Did" questions should be mixed (as is shown on the following page).

Beginning Reading Comprehension: Who? and What did (or do)?

Circle the word(s) that answers the question.

1. The (boy) walked   Who walked? _____

   _____

2. (Dad) talked.   Who talked? _____

   _____

3. The (baby) cried.   Who cried? _____

   _____

4. The (girl) jumped.   Who jumped? _____

   _____

Pre-Reading Comprehension: Who? and What did (or do)?

The child should read the sentence and then answer the question by circling the word in the sentence that answers the "Who" question. Next, the child should underline the word in the sentence that answers the "Did What?" question. Then, the child can draw a line connecting the noun with WHO, or the verb with the WHAT. This level of the exercise combines both "Who" and "What Did" questions in a mixed order. The therapist should keep producing new sheets in the same format (mixed questions, different persons - pronouns, noun, and proper nouns) until the child can easily complete the sheet him/herself. Once the child can complete the sheet without the therapist's prompts, it is time to start higher level reading comprehension activities (which follow).

Beginning Reading Comprehension: Who? and What did (or do)?

Circle the word(s) that answers the Who question and underline the word that answers the What question. Then connect the answers to the questions with a line.

1. The (boy) walked   What did the boy do?
    Who walked?

2. (Dad) talked.   Who talked?
    What did dad do?

3. The (baby) cried.   Who cried?
    What did the baby do?

4. The (girl) jumped.   What did the girl do?
    Who jumped?

How To Do Reading Comprehension

The reading comprehension activity is very involved. Therefore, it is important that the therapist go step by step and read the complete section before introducing the exercise to the child. The stories chosen must be beginning comprehension stories. It is important that even the easiest stories have a **simple sequence** of events. Reading Milestones has a series that works well with the reading comprehension exercise.

Note: Reading Milestones (1991 Dormac Inc.) can be ordered through:

Edmark, P.O. Box 3218, Redmond WA 98073-3218
(800) 362-2890.

1. First, the therapist must pre-read the story and prepare the "mixed up order" on the STORY SEQUENCE sheet. It is crucial that the main, important events pertaining to the sequence of the story be included on the sheet. A detail such as "the hat was red" is not good to use for sequencing.

2. Next, the child must be shown the title of the story and the picture on the title page or book cover. Have him/her predict what the story is about. The therapist should say: "What do you think the story is about?" The child's idea needs to be written down on the STORY REPORT form along with the title and author (if there is an author).

3. The therapist should have the child read the story aloud. The child should be told to stop every couple of pages so the therapist can help him/her identify new characters and list the most important events that happen (what is selected should mirror what the therapist prepared in the "mixed order" sequence). The child's answers should be recorded on the "Important Story Events" sheet. When finished, the child should be prompted to verbally explain the story using the "Important Story Events" sheet as a cue. Once the child can verbally explain the story using the sheet, then the child should be required to tell the story without the sheet as a cue.

4. After the child has finished the story, the therapist should have him/her complete any work sheets that might accompany the story (e.g. Reading Milestones Comprehension work sheets).

5. Next, the mixed order -> correct order story sequence should be completed with the child. The therapist must explain that "this is the wrong/mixed up order. What is the right order? What happened first...", etc.

6. Then, the therapist should help the child complete the "Story Report" form which asks questions about the story e.g. It WAS about: Who?, Where?, What Happened?

7. Last, the therapist should have the child complete the "Story Summary" form. The therapist must make sure that the child summarizes the story in the correct sequential order.

8. An advanced variation of this is to have the child read the mixed order -> correct order story sequence and have the child summarize the story using the Summarizing form.

This activity takes a long time (perhaps over an hour). Ideally, the child should work on one story a week, reviewing the sequence of the story daily. Reviewing does NOT include redoing all exercises. The therapist should ask the relevant WH questions (Who, Where, and What Happened) and questions about the sequence. Despite the large amount of time that this exercise set takes, it will show the therapist where the child's deficits are in terms of sequencing, summarizing, and general story comprehension. If done regularly, changes in the child's ability to comprehend simple stories should be seen relatively quickly.

Why Do Comprehension Drills?

Children with pervasive developmental disorders are often good at decoding sentences; however, they have great difficulty in comprehending what they are reading. Part of the difficulty comes from the inability to sequence well and having a limited vocabulary. These reading comprehension activities are designed 1) to make the structure of stories explicit and 2) to help strengthen the child's ability to sequence. Story comprehension is the one of the most difficult type of language-related skills for these children. Therefore, it is a good idea to work on fictional reading comprehension once the child can comfortably decode simple text (for many children this occurs in first grade).

Important Story Events

This is the first of 4 sheets that can be used when teaching reading comprehension. This first sheet has the child name all the characters and tell what happened. The therapist should have the child stop reading every few lines to fill in this sheet. *Note: The example used in this sheet is quite high level. The story read was taken from the 5th book of 10 in level 3 of Reading Milestones. Typically, the child should start with a much lower level story.*

Important Story Events	
Title: In the Cookie House	

Characters (Who)	Sequence of Events (What Happens)
Gretel	nuts ground.
Hansel	went to sleep
Mom	walked far woods
Dad	ate cookie house
Sandman	locked the door
Witch	pushed witch oven
	hugged

Story Sequence

This is the second of 4 sheets that should be used when teaching reading comprehension. The second sheet requires the child take all the major events in the story and put them in the correct order. This is a particularly important skill for the child to master since ability to sequence is inextricably linked to story comprehension. It is important that the therapist write up the mixed order of story events before beginning the entire comprehension exercise with the child.

Story Sequence

Title: In the Cookie House

Mixed Up Order	Right Order
Mom and Dad found Hansel and Gretel.	Hansel and Gretel found nuts on the ground.
They walked far into the woods.	They walked far into the woods.
The bad old witch put Hansel in a room.	Hansel and Gretel tasted the cookie house.
Gretel pushed the witch into the oven.	The bad old witch put Hansel in a room.
Hansel and Gretel tasted the cookie house.	Gretel pushed the witch into the oven.
Hansel and Gretel found nuts on the ground.	Mom and Dad found Hansel and Gretel.

What happened first? Hansel and Gretel found some nuts.

What happened last? Mom and Dad found Hansel and Gretel.

Story Report

This is the third of 4 sheets that should be used when teaching reading comprehension. The third sheet requires the child to report on the story by asking him/her to answer assorted important questions about the story such as Who, Where, and What Happened. The structure created by this form helps clarify the story to the child. This sheet will help the child throughout his/her schooling since the child will be asked to read and report on books in several grades.

Story Report

DATE:

TITLE OF THE BOOK: _____ In the Cookie House _____

AUTHOR:_____

My prediction: I think the book is about _____ a gingerbread house. There is a gingerbread man. The cookie house is sweet.

IT WAS ABOUT:

     WHO? Hansel, Gretel, Mom, Dad, Witch, Sandman.

     WHERE? in the cookie house

     WHAT HAPPENED?

FIRST Hansel and Gretel found some nuts on the ground.

THEN they ate the candy house.

LAST Dad and Mom and Hansel and Gretel hugged.

WHAT I LIKED ABOUT THE BOOK: I liked the book because I liked the sweet house.

Story Summary

This is the fourth sheet in the series that can be used when teaching reading comprehension. This form has the child briefly summarize the story in a structured way. This last sheet tells the therapist how much of the story was understood. If the child is not able to comprehend the story (as evidenced by this last sheet), then the next story chosen should be much shorter and at a lower level using the same four sheet system.

Story Summary

The story___In the Cookie House___takes

place ___in the sweet candy house___. The main

character s are Hansel and Gretel who___ate the___

sweet house.___.

In this story___Dad and Mom walked into the___

woods to find Hansel and Gretel.___

___

At the end, ___Dad and Mom hugged Hansel and___

Gretel.___

___

Summarizing Independently

When the child is able to complete the 3 or 4 forms that precede the Story Summary sheet, then s/he should be given the opportunity to independently complete this form. This is a very advanced skill since it works on an important deficit - sequencing - which is very difficult for so many language delayed children. Once the child completes this form, he should then be required to verbally summarize the story without the form.

Summarizing Independently

Read the story sequence. Tell what the story is about.

The story is about Hansel and Gretel who went to the
cookie house.

They found some nuts to eat.

They went to the woods.

They ate a piece of the gingerbread house

The witch found them.

They put the witch into the oven.

Mom and Dad Found Hansel and Gretel.

Reading Comprehension Record

This sheet is designed to keep track of the stories and exercises completed with each story. If one person is in charge of the reading comprehension, this record is not critical; however, if a number of people are working with the child, it is important to keep a record of the stories completed so that 1) there is no duplication and 2) the child does all the exercises appropriate for his/her level (this will vary from child to child). This record is designed to be used by therapists, not by the child.

The exercises listed on the left of the Reading Comprehension Record are less advanced than those listed on the right.

Reading Comprehension Record

Story: _Hansel and Gretel_   Date started: _6/22/96_
      Book: _Book 5, Level 3_
- ☒ Predict What the Story is About
- ☒ Read the Story   ☐ Summarize Independently
- ☒ Do the Important Story Events Sheet ☐ Take Notes from the Story
- ☒ Do Work Sheets (that may accompany the story)
- ☒ Do Story Sequence Sheet (Mixed Order - Correct Order)
- ☒ Do Story Report Sheet
- ☒ Do Story Summary Sheet   ☐ Make an Outline of the Story
                                ☐ Write a Descriptive Paragraph Based on Part of the Story

Notes: _____   Date Completed: _6/29/96_
_____

Story: _The Three Little Pigs_   Date started: _6/30/96_
      Book: _Book 5, Level 3_
- ☒ Predict What the Story is About
- ☒ Read the Story   ☐ Summarize Independently
- ☒ Do the Important Story Events Sheet ☐ Take Notes from the Story
- ☒ Do Work Sheets (that may accompany the story)
- ☒ Do Story Sequence Sheet (Mixed Order - Correct Order)
- ☒ Do Story Report Sheet
- ☒ Do Story Summary Sheet   ☐ Make an Outline of the Story
                                ☐ Write a Descriptive Paragraph Based on Part of the Story

Notes: _____   Date Completed: _7/06/96_
_____

Story: _Little Red Riding Hood_   Date started: _7/07/96_
      Book: _Book 5, Level 3_
- ☒ Predict What the Story is About
- ☒ Read the Story   ☐ Summarize Independently
- ☒ Do the Important Story Events Sheet ☐ Take Notes from the Story
- ☒ Do Work Sheets (that may accompany the story)
- ☒ Do Story Sequence Sheet (Mixed Order - Correct Order)
- ☒ Do Story Report Sheet
- ☒ Do Story Summary Sheet   ☐ Make an Outline of the Story
                                ☐ Write a Descriptive Paragraph Based on Part of the Story

Notes: _____   Date Completed: _7/14/96_
_____

Further Comprehension Activities

These two activities concentrate on reading comprehension in different ways. The first activity, "Identifying the Kind of Text Read" has the child find clues as to the kind of paragraph or story s/he will read. The second activity, "Event or Detail", has the child identify whether the sentence or phrase is important to the comprehension of the story, or simply a detail that makes the story more complete or colorful. Both these drills should be done only when the child is proficient at the Reading Comprehension Activities that precede this section.

1. Identifying the Kind of Text Read

The therapist has the child look at each title. From the words in the title the child must identify whether the title is from a STORY, a DESCRIPTIVE/FACTUAL paragraph, a COMPARATIVE paragraph or a "HOW TO" paragraph. The therapist must begin with obvious "How To" paragraphs (where the words "How To" are in the title), or factual paragraphs (where the topic is mentioned in the title). Obvious story titles to begin with are those that state explicitly in the title the subject and the verb e.g. "John goes skating", or "Sally rides her bike." Only when the child is proficient at the obvious titles should it be made more challenging using such titles as "The Snowy Day". This title could easily confuse a child since the s/he may think that the book is about weather. Eventually, the child will learn that some titles are ambiguous and that the best way to find out the type of paragraph or book is to read the first paragraph.

2. Event or Detail

The therapist has the child look at the sentence and decide whether it is a detail or an event that is important to the paragraph. This is difficult because a statement can be either an event or detail depending upon how it relates to the story, and not on the intrinsic content of the sentence itself. This is a good drill to introduce once the child has completed many reading comprehension sheet series (presented earlier in the chapter) and understands a specific story quite well. Only then should details and events from that story be presented to the child for him/her to discern event from detail.

Why Teach These Drills?

Reading comprehension is a multifaceted problem for children with language disorders. The key to attacking this deficit is to use a variety of tactics. These two exercises are presented with this philosophy in mind. The "Identifying the Kind of Text" activity is designed to teach the child key words which give the reader the idea of what kind of text to expect. The "Event or Detail" activity uses phrase types and phrase order to help the child define the sentence as important or unimportant.

Identifying the Kind of Text Read

This sheet is designed to teach the child to identify the type of text that s/he is reading. This is an important skill because it will determine how the child goes about understanding the text. For example, if the text is a story, then sequence is important; whereas, if the text is factual, there is often no real sequence to understand.

Identifying the Kind of Text Read

Date: _____

Look at each title. Tell whether the title tells you if what is read will be a STORY, a DESCRIPTIVE/FACTUAL paragraph, a COMPARATIVE paragraph or a "HOW TO" paragraph.

Title	Type of Paragraph(s)/Text
Forests	Descriptive/factual
Molly's Day at School	Story
The Solar System	Descriptive/factual
Joe's Vacation	Story

Give an example of a title for a story, descriptive/factual paragraph, comparative paragraph, or "how to" paragraph:

Oceans

Molly's Day at the Park

Event or Detail?

This exercise is designed to teach the child to identify whether the sentence describes an event or a detail in the story. This is an important skill because if the child concentrates on each sentence of the story equally, it will be very hard to comprehend the story. **The child needs to be told and remember that an action is always an event, and a description is always a detail.** The therapist should ask: Why is this an event? (because it happened). Why is this a detail? (because it is a description).

Event or Detail?

Read each sentence from a story. Tell whether it is an event of the story or a detail. Then recall one more event and one more detail from the story.

Story: __Pocahontas__   Event or Detail?

Pocahontas was an Indian   __Detail__

John Smith met Pocahontas   __Event__

Pocahontas had black hair   __Detail__

John Smith's boat was big   __Detail__

Event in: __Pocahontas__   Pocahontas talked to Grand-

mother Willow.

Detail in: __Pocahontas__   The Indians picked

corn.

How To Teach Math Word Problems

Prerequisite: In order for a child to work on math word problems, s/he should have a firm grasp of simple addition. **If the child does not have this skill, the child must be taught to count and add before this activity is introduced.**

Once the child understands simple addition, the next step is to teach the child to write a math word problem. The first math problems should be written for addition only, and the therapist should use very low numbers. The four key words used in addition problems are: "'in all", "all together", "total number" and "in total". The therapist should choose one of these four key words for each math word problem. At first, the therapist will have to prompt the child heavily through this drill, since the child probably has never been introduced to math word problems before. After a few math problems have been written with the child, s/he will understand the structure of a math addition problem and should have no trouble writing one. It is important to keep in mind that this exercise is to improve the child's reading comprehension, not his/her math skills.

Given the number, equation and key words, the first step is to have the child write the problem about a subject of his/her choice. For example, the child may choose "lollipops eaten". Once the child truly understands the pattern of a math word problem (which should not take long), then the therapist can make this drill harder by choosing the object and the verb. For example, the child may choose the verb eaten; however, if the therapist chooses the object and verb "goals scored", the child must work harder to write the problem because the child may not know how to conjugate the verb "scored". In this manner, this drill develops the child's ability to conjugate verbs. In addition, the therapist can further constrain the word problem by choosing the subject of the problem i.e. John, Judy, the kids. In this way the child must make the name of the child agree with the pronoun. Furthermore, the therapist can introduce the word "more", so the child knows that when additional items are added, "how many MORE" is the way to ask the addition question. As long as the child's peers are working on addition at school, the child should create <u>addition</u> word problems.

The child always composes the word problem although the therapist writes it down. Then, the child can write the answer him/herself. Children generally find answering the math word problem reinforcing, since they find writing the problem the more challenging task.

Subtraction word problems are done in exactly the same way except that the key words are different. The key words for subtraction are: left, remain, and difference. The question is: "How many _____ are left" or "remain" or "What is the difference?" An example of a subtraction word problem is: "Jane had 6 apples. She GAVE 3 apples away. How many apples were left."

Multiplication word problems are done in exactly the same way except that the key words are the same as addition. The key words for multiplication are: "in all", "all together", "total number" and "in total." And the question is: "How many _____ are there (in all, all together, in total)?, or What is the total number of _____?" An example of a multiplication word problem is: "Jane had two apple barrels with two apples in each barrel. How many apples were there all together?"

Division word problems are done in exactly the same way except that the key words are different. The key words for division are: "in each _____" or "each ___ get." And the question is: "How many _____ does each (person, group, pile etc.) get?" An example of a division problem is: "Joan had 6 apples. She split them into 3 piles. How many apples were in each pile."

NOTE: The therapist should NOT assume that the child understands this drill if they can answer the question. If this drill seems to be too easy, the therapist should make it more difficult rather than stop having the child do it. Ways of increasing difficulty are:
   1. to add more people to the problem
   2. to constrain the word problems by requiring certain objects and verbs

Last Steps:

1. Answering math word problems orally
The child should be able to eventually answer a math problem presented to her/him orally ONLY. Once the child can correctly answer a math word problem with no visual prompts, then it is clear that the child truly understands the concept of math word problems.

2. Asking math word problems orally
This is also a good drill to do with children who have mastered word problems. The therapist should ask the child to create a word problem without allowing him/her to write it out first. This will require heavy prompting at first; the goal is to have the child be able to create a word problem with no visual cues.

Why Teach Children To Write Math Problems?

Children with developmental disorders are often very good at recognizing and figuring out patterns. Consequently, mathematics is often an area in which these children excel. However, they can have a great deal of difficulty when mathematical concepts are combined with language in the form of word problems. Therefore, it is important that they learn to identify the parts of language which convey what kind of problem is being asked. The child generated word problem activity works on this ability.

In addition, by requiring these children to write their own math problems, the therapist is able to work on comprehension, verb tense and noun/pronoun agreement. For example, the child must learn that if "John has 5 balloons and someone gives him 5 balloons", **him** is related to the word John. Another example of agreement is "John has", and "someone gives", and "How many balloons does John have".

Furthermore, word problems are often a highly motivating way to practice various skills since children who are good at math and patterns enjoy this exercise.

Math Word Problems

The Math Problem exercise is designed to teach reading comprehension by pairing words to symbols. Once the child has learned the key words for addition, then the key words for subtraction can be taught. Math word problems are a particular challenge for children with language disorders even if they are good at math. This exercise makes math problems easier to understand and complete.

Math Problems

Number Equation   **Key Word(s)**

1 + 5   games
                 played   in all

Word Problem: _John played one game with_

Kate. Then he played 5 more games with Jim. How

many games did he play in all? **6 games**

Number Equation   **Key Word(s)**

3 + 4   cookies
                 eaten   all together

Word Problem: _Jane ate 3 cookies. Then_

she ate 4 more cookies. How many cookies did she

eat all together? **7 cookies**

How To Increase Concepts Through Vocabulary

New Vocabulary Introduction

New Vocabulary Sheet
The first step to increasing vocabulary is to teach the child how to define the meanings of words s/he already knows. For example, the therapist should start with a word that the child is interested in such as "Balloon". The child is required to 1) define the balloon (with heaving prompting), 2) give the therapist a number of things one can do with a balloon, and 3) give a list of a number of different places one could find a balloon. As the child improves at this drill, the lists could change to other things such as "things a balloon has" or "people who use a balloon" or "describe a balloon". Once the lists are completed, then the child must use the word in three separate sentences. After the initial word definition exercise, the child should be required to take the new word and use it in two separate and novel sentences during subsequent therapy sessions. By the end of the week, the child will probably be able to define that word well. A maximum of two words per week should be introduced. Eventually (when the child is able to define many of the words he knows in this manner), then the vocabulary sheet can be used to introduce new words. An easy child's dictionary is good to have so the child can find a definition of a new word being introduced. If the child easily understands how to define words s/he knows, the therapist should begin to introduce novel words. This is a good exercise to teach synonyms. For example, the child may know what a bear is, but not what a cub is.

Once the child can define words using the sheet, it is time to for the therapist to introduce the next exercise (for most children this will take a very long time).

Orally Defining Objects, People and Verbs
This advanced new vocabulary introduction has the child define new words in a very constrained way. Once the child defines the word, s/he must put the word into three sentences, one relating to home, one relating to school, and one relating to the community. This vocabulary drill cannot be introduced until the child has learned in depth about the meaning of "community (from Chapter 3). *Note: Not all words lend themselves to this format; therefore, the therapist must make sure that the word chosen is going to work before it is introduced to the child.*

New Vocabulary Synonyms - Easy

The next vocabulary exercise has the child learn about synonyms and usage. The therapist writes a new word the child has learned from the vocabulary sheet described above, and the child writes the synonym that they already know. Then the child is prompted to put the new word into a sentence in much the same way as was done in the first vocabulary drill sheet.

New Vocabulary Synonyms - Difficult

Once the child has learned 5 or so new words (over a couple of weeks), then the therapist should create a paragraph using those five words. The therapist circles the new words and the child is required to write the synonym or a short definition above the circled word. Then the child should be instructed to reread the paragraph using the synonyms.

Using New Vocabulary - Stories

The next activity to be introduced has the child use the new vocabulary to create a VERY short story. The therapist must give the child three words and a title for the story. The child must create one sentence for each new word. Each sentence must somehow relate to the other (either through a main character or main event).

Applying New Vocabulary

This sheet has the child apply each vocabulary word in different settings in order to make sure the child understands the definition and how the word is to be used. This activity assumes that the child has already learned about community from Chapter 3.

New Vocabulary For The Week

This sheet has the child state what kind of word the new word is (a descriptive word, or a noun, or verb for example), and has the child give a synonym or definition, and an application of the word. This is an advanced vocabulary exercise.

New Vocabulary To Be Reinforced

This sheet keeps a record of all the vocabulary introduced, some of which may need periodic reinforcing. This list is designed for the therapy record, not for the child to work from directly.

Why Work On Increasing Vocabulary?

Children with auditory processing problems do not pick up vocabulary FROM THE NATURAL ENVIRONMENT at the same rate as do typically developing children. These children do not generally ask questions about a word they have heard but do not understand. Therefore, it is imperative that children with developmental disorders learn to pick up vocabulary from both the natural environment and other sources such as books. These exercises are designed to introduce the child to word meanings and definitions, give him/her the tools to define words independently, and therefore, be able to understand definitions when presented to them by others or through dictionaries and encyclopedias.

New Vocabulary

This exercise teaches new noun vocabulary and works on the concept that words can be defined. First, the child should be instructed to define the word. Then, the therapist should choose two descriptions and have the child give suggestions as to the function of the object or give a description of the object. It is important to introduce words the child already knows since the skill to be learned is defining words or understanding that words have definitions. Later, words that the child does not know can be introduced with the use of this sheet and a child's dictionary.

New Vocabulary

Descriptions e.g. things you can do with a _tree_ ; where you see a _____; who has a _____, what goes in a _____, etc...

Tree :	**is a plant.**
(New word)	
	(Definition of new word)

Descriptions e.g. things you can do with a _tree_ ; where you see a _____; who has a ____ , what goes in a, etc....

What do you do with a tree?	Describe a tree.
climb	flowers
pick oranges	bush
pick apples	trunk
pick snails	branches
look at it	leaves
sit under it	nest
stand up under it	brown
	green

New word used in sentences:

I climbed the tree.
I pick snails off the tree.
I sit under the tree.

Orally Defining Words (Objects)

This vocabulary exercise gives the child the opportunity to learn to define objects by what they do or by which group they belong to. Then, the sheet instructs the child to use the word in sentences relating to a variety of settings. This sheet should not be introduced to the child until the child has finished the Community script in Chapter 3. Once the child has completed the form, s/he should define the word, first using the form as a visual cue, and then, without the form.

Orally Defining Words (Objects)

Title: _____ball_____

Description	Group	Use
Tell something about it; it?		**What do you do with**
round	toy	bounces
_____		

Definition: A ___ball___ is a ___round toy___ that

___bounces___

Sentences

Home: I play ball in the back yard.

School: I play ball at recess with Josh.

Community: I went to a baseball game with Dad.

Orally Defining Words (People)

This vocabulary exercise gives the child the opportunity to learn to define people by what they are and by which group they belong to. Then, the sheet instructs the child to use the word in a sentence as it relates to a variety of settings. This sheet should not be introduced to the child until the child has finished the Community script in Chapter 3. The child should orally define the word, first using the sheet and then, without the sheet.

Orally Defining Words (People)

Title: _boy_

Description	**Group**	**Is/Has/Does**
Use male or female		
male	person	child

Definition: A _boy_ **is a** _male person_ **that**

Sentences _is a child._

Home: _A boy lives in a house._

School: _A boy does math at school._

Community: _A boy likes to go to the YMCA._

Orally Defining Words (Verbs)

This vocabulary exercise gives the child the opportunity to learn to define verbs by what they are for (their purpose) and which body part one does them with. Then the sheet has the child use the word in sentences relating to a variety of settings. This sheet should not be introduced to the child until the child has finished the Community script in Chapter 3. The child should orally define the word, first using the sheet and then, without the sheet.

Orally Defining Words (Verbs)

Title: _run_

Verb/Action	**Done with**	**Purpose**
	body part or object	lets you ...
Running	_feet_	_go places_

Definition: _Running_ **is something you do with**

your feet **to** _go places._

Sentences

Home: _I like to run in the backyard._

School: _I run in P.E. on the sports field._

Community: _I like to run at the park._

Vocabulary and Synonyms - Easy

This new vocabulary exercise requires the child to use all the words s/he has learned through the new vocabulary sheets by finding a word that means the same thing and then using the word in a sentence. This should be done with the words that have been introduced through the new vocabulary sheets. This should NOT be done with any words that have not been introduced in this way since it will be very difficult for the child to come up with synonyms by him/herself without knowing the definition of a word.

Synonyms

Write down a synonym - a word that means the same thing as the word listed. Then use the new word in a sentence.

New Word - Synonym	Sentence
cub - baby bear	I saw a cub.
beautiful - pretty	The girl was beautiful.
lawn - grass	The lawn is green.
soil - dirt	Plants grow in soil.
exhausted - very tired	Mom was exhausted.
tiny - little	The baby was tiny.

Vocabulary and Synonyms - Difficult

This is a sample of a paragraph given to a child to work on synonyms . It is important to write stories that will interest the child.

Synonyms

Write a synonym or definition above each circled word in the story.

The Bear family lived in a big tree house in the

woods

baby bear

(forest.) One day, Mama Bear was watching her (cub)

play outside. The cub was doing somersaults on the

grass   *soft*

front (lawn.) The sun was very warm and the (fluffy)

beautiful

clouds in the sky looked (magnificent.) Mama Bear

dirt

was busy shoveling (soil) in her garden. She was

tired

working very hard and felt (exhausted.) When she

little

finished digging, Mama Bear planted many (tiny) seeds

in the ground. She was growing corn in her garden.

Using New Vocabulary: Stories

This vocabulary exercise gives the child the opportunity to use the words s/he has learned in a story. Through this exercise, the child learns that those words found in a story are relevant and can be used in other stories. In addition, this exercise strengthens the child's comprehension of the word so that when the child sees the word in a new story, s/he will understand it.

Using New Vocabulary In Stories

Use these words in a short story: <u>soil, magnificent, exhausted</u>

TITLE: _____<u>The Home</u>_____

PROMPTS:

Who	Did What	When	Why

<u>The bear made a magnificent</u>

<u>house in the soil. He was</u>

<u>exhausted. Then he went to</u>

<u>sleep.</u>

_____

_____

Applying New Vocabulary

The Applying New Vocabulary exercise requires the child to use all the words s/he has learned through the new vocabulary sheets in three different settings. This should be done with <u>all</u> applicable words that have been introduced through the new vocabulary exercises.

Applying New Vocabulary

Tell how you would apply or use each word at home, at school, or out in the community

Word	Home	School	Community
cup	I drink from a cup at dinner.	I do not use a cup at school.	I drink from a cup at the restaurant,
scissors	John cuts paper with scissors at home.	I cut with scissors in art at school.	The hair dresser uses scissors to cut my hair.
chair	I sit in a chair when I watch videos.	I sit in a chair at my desk at school.	I sit in a chair at the movie theater.

New Vocabulary for the Week

This exercise has the child provide a synonym for the weekly words (thereby defining the word), identify the kind of word it is (its function) and apply the word in any way the child is able. This is a much more difficult vocabulary exercise than the previous exercises since it concentrates on the skills used in several drills. When the child can easily complete the easier vocabulary drills, this drill should be introduced and done with <u>all</u> new vocabulary words introduced to the child. This exercise should NOT be done with any words that have not been introduced through the other exercises.

New Vocabulary for the Week

1. Define the word.
2. Write down what kind of word it is.
3. Write down where or how you would use the word.

Word	Definition	Kind of Word	Where/ How Might Use/ Apply the Word	
<u>tiny</u>	small +	describes	some tiny things <u>at home</u> <u>at school</u> beads eraser corn candy	
<u>pleased</u>	happy +	describes	who can be pleased mom dad grandma	When they are pleased when I act nice when I sing softly when I play piano

New Vocabulary To Be Reinforced

This vocabulary sheet is provided as a therapy record to keep track of all the vocabulary words that have been recently introduced. This is not a form the child should work with.

New Vocabulary To Be Reinforced

New Word - Definition or Word Paired With	New Word - Definition or Word Paired With
cub - baby bear	
lawn - grass	
soil - dirt	
exhausted - very tired	
tiny - little	
search - look for	
vanished - was gone	
evening - early night	
started - began	
silent - very quiet	
leaped - jumped	
gigantic - big	
sparkling - shining	
pleased - happy	
hiked - walked	

How To Teach Sequencing

Children with developmental disorders generally have one major deficit in common: they are unable to sequence. By sequencing, we mean that the child has not grasped the concept that everything happens in relation to everything else.   They will have no problem memorizing the sequence of things and they will be able to recite ordered information very well e.g. the alphabet, numbers; however, the concept of sequence is not understood.   This is one of the reasons why these children have problems comprehending stories or particular concepts. Unfortunately, sequencing is related to many abstract concepts. At first glance, most parents will believe that this is not the case with their child; however, the following drills will help indicate the deficit and work to minimize the problem.

The following drills are designed to attack the sequencing problem from the deficit. The major areas in which sequencing plays an important role are numbers, calendar, time, money, daily routines, and activity routines. This book offers materials and drills to work on each area in a slow, methodical manner.   The order that these concepts are taught correspond to when the concepts are typically introduced. This will depend upon several factors including the child's age and ability, as well as when the child's peers learn these skills.

Sequencing Concepts

1. Sequencing of Numbers
It is important that the basic principles of number sequencing be taught first. This is the easiest form of sequencing, often introduced in kindergarten if not earlier. The more complex concepts such as Place Value should not be introduced until taught in school.

2. Calendar
 Once the child grasps number sequencing, then basic calendar skills must be taught (this is taught in kindergarten, through grade two). When calendar is first introduced, the child should be taught simply to identify the day, date, month and year (which is written on the calendar) in much the same way as is taught in kindergarten. This level of the skill is sufficient for kindergarten. Once the child is in first grade and on, it is time to teach calendar in a more in depth manner (outlined in the section on Calendar). A deep understanding of calendar may take a long time to learn; therefore, calendar should be a short part of every therapy session.

3. Time
The ability to tell time is taught in kindergarten and first grade. The child should be taught to tell time when his/her peers learn it. Telling time, however, is different from understanding time. Once the child is good at telling time, only then is it a good idea to start teaching about time, based on the time teaching hierarchy outlined in this chapter. Time is another concept that may take years for many children to grasp. Therefore, this skill should be revisited frequently, with higher level time concepts introduced gradually.

How To Teach Sequencing (Continued)

4. Money

Money is often introduced in first grade, and is used throughout elementary school. It is important to introduce the basics of money in first grade; however, money is an abstract concept that needs to be taught in many different ways in order for the child to be able to competently handle money. See the section on Money in this chapter for more detailed information on how to teach the concept of money.

5. Sequencing of Daily Events

The sequencing of daily events can be taught any time after numbers are taught. This skill is important and should be worked on daily.

6. Sequencing of Activities

The sequencing of activities can be taught any time after numbers and daily events are taught. The simple sequencing of an activity helps the child with the concept that there is an ordering in time to everything we do.

 If the drills are not taught slowly and in the correct order (according to the hierarchies that are laid out in the various sections), it is very difficult for even the brightest child to succeed since the drills in each section are sequenced from simple to complex. IT IS VERY IMPORTANT NOT TO SKIP AROUND QUICKLY FROM CONCEPT TO CONCEPT. It should be noted that some children never completely grasp sequencing. Even a partial grasp of the concept provides a foundation for other language-based concepts and is, therefore, important to teach.

Most of the concepts are introduced with a script that is read with the child. The therapist reads a sentence and then the child reads a sentence, alternating through the script. Then, the equations that accompany the script are read by the child and therapist. The adult who works through the script with the child should read the entire section on each concept prior to introducing the concept to make sure that the concept is introduced according to the instructions given. It is also important that the adult go slowly through these concepts in order to avoid confusion for the child.

NOTE: Time and Money will take a long time to teach; therefore, it is suggested that they not both be introduced at the same time. Once the child has a beginner's understanding of one concept, then the other concept can be introduced.

Why Teach Sequencing?

Sequencing must be taught because it is all pervasive. A lack of understanding of this concept will interfere with the child's ability to learn about time and money which are integral to future independence as well as adversely affect the child's ability to comprehend much information presented through books, television and in person in a large group. In short, sequencing is a cornerstone of language comprehension.

How To Teach Sequencing With Numbers

The first step in teaching sequencing with numbers is to see whether the child can put numbers in order from 1 to 100. This is a different skill from the child being able to count to 100. The therapist should have the child sequence numbers from 1) smallest to largest, 2) largest to smallest, 3) lowest number to highest number, 4) highest number to lowest number. Once the child can do the above, it is time to introduce the Ordering Information activity sheet.

Using the Ordering Information Drill
The therapist should have the child sequence numbers, ages, and people (in terms of age). Once the child becomes proficient at numbers and ages, then the Sequencing and Ordering sheet can be introduced.

Using the Sequencing and Ordering Drill
The therapist should prepare the Sequencing and Ordering Sheets with numbers and ages. The child should number the ages or numbers from 1) youngest to oldest, 2) oldest to youngest , 3) highest to lowest, and 4) lowest to highest. Once the child can sequence and order numbers and ages using this exercise, the Comparing Numbers exercise can be introduced.

Comparing Numbers Exercise
The Comparing Numbers exercise is designed to reinforce the earlier drills . The child should circle the higher, bigger, lower or smaller number depending on the specifications set by the therapist on the sheet. Note that bigger and biggest is not introduced at this point.

Understanding Place Value
This exercise should be introduced only if the child's typically developing peers are learning or have learned this skill. The therapist should introduce the place value script heavily prompting the child to give the right answer by having the child count the digits and then prompting the child to say what each column means. Once the child understands the pattern, the prompts should be faded.

Why Teach Sequencing With Numbers?

Sequencing is a very important skill that is critical to understand in reading comprehension, mathematics, using money, telling time and truly understanding the calendar. Therefore, it is a good idea to concentrate on this skill from a variety of different angles. Sequencing with numbers is the most basic form of sequencing and the easiest for most children to understand. Therefore, we begin with number sequencing prior to introducing most other skills that require sequencing.

Ordering Information

This exercise has the child order information given in a specified sequence. In this example, the therapist gives all the information out of order and the child is required to number the information according to the instructions.

Ordering Information

Follow each direction. Put the items in order. Use a 1 (first), 2 (second), 3 (third) order.

1. Order these _people_ from _oldest_ to _youngest_

    1   mommy

    3   Susie

    2   David

2. Order these _ages_ from _youngest_ to _oldest_

    1   2 years old

    3 55 years old

    2 16 years old

3. Order these _people_ from _oldest_ to _youngest_

    3   John, age 5

    1   Mark, age 65

    2 Lindsay, age 7

Sequencing and Ordering

This exercise, like the one before it, has the child order the information given in a specified sequence. In this example, the therapist concentrates on the concept of relative age. This exercise can also be used with numbers.

Sequencing and Ordering

Read each direction and order the ___ages___ by writing 1 2, 3, and 4 in the correct boxes.

youngest to oldest   12 years   62 years   5 years   26 years

        2   4   1   3

oldest to youngest   10 years   35 years   19 years   44 years

        4   2   3   1

youngest to oldest   1 year   23 years   8 years   36 years

        1   3   2   4

oldest to youngest   2 years   53 years   89 years   3 years

        4   2   1   3

Comparing Numbers

This exercise provides a way to practice skills gained in the number sequencing and ordering drills. The Comparing Numbers exercise is also another way to strengthen new knowledge the child has gained about place value and sequencing (which follows).

Comparing Numbers

Look at each number. Count the number of digits in each number. Circle the number that is bigger or smaller, higher or lower.

HIGHEST	22	(250)	5
BIGGEST	(108)	96	103
LOWEST	22	(8)	34
SMALLEST	100	1000	(10)
LOWEST	(19)	219	421

Write a number that is _lower_ than ___188___ . _8_

Write a number that is _bigger_ than ___100___ . 250

Write a number that is _smaller_ than ___65___ . 4

Write a number that is _higher_ than ___212___ . 233

Place Value (Introduction)

If the child is learning math in a mainstream environment, the place value script should be introduced when the child's typically developing peers are introduced to it and not before. If mainstreaming is not a concern, then the child may learn this script only on a "need to know" basis since place value is quite an advanced skill (even at the introductory level).

Place Value (Introduction)

ALL NUMBERS are made up of **DIGITS.**

A **DIGIT** is any **NUMBER FROM 0 to 9.**

SOME NUMBERS have more **DIGITS** than other numbers.

If a number has **MORE DIGITS** than another number, it is a **BIGGER NUMBER.** It is a **HIGHER NUMBER.**

Its **AMOUNT IS MORE THAN THE OTHER NUMBER.**

The number 10 has more **DIGITS** than the number 5.

The number 10 has two **DIGITS.** The number 5 has one **DIGIT.**

The number 10 is a **BIGGER NUMBER** than the number 5.

The number 1,000 has four **DIGITS.** The number 532 has three **DIGITS.**

The number 1,000 is a **HIGHER NUMBER** than the number 532.

Each **DIGIT** in a number is **EQUAL TO A SPECIAL AMOUNT.**

You need to **LOOK AT THE PLACE** where a **DIGIT** is found in a number to tell the **SPECIAL AMOUNT** it equals.

The **SPECIAL AMOUNT** that each **DIGIT** equals depends on the **PLACE VALUE** of the **DIGIT.**

Here is the **VALUE** of each digit's **PLACE** in a number.

This will tell you about the **PLACE VALUE** of a **DIGIT.**

To make these last two lines meaningful, point to the Place Value in the following Diagram.

Place Value Continued (Introduction)

The visual representation of place value should be introduced concurrently with the script since this graphic is a visual representation of what is explained in the script.

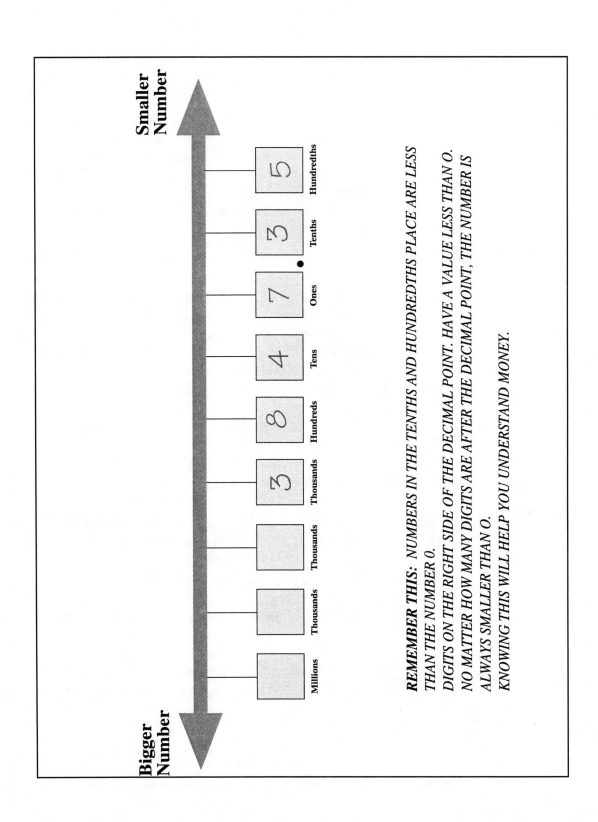

More About Place Value (Advanced)

Before this script is introduced, the child must have mastered the introductory place value script. Again, it is important to know the level of understanding of complex place value concepts among the child's typically developing peers. Place value should be explained to the child so that s/he will not fall behind rather than tutor the child privately so that s/he will be far ahead of his/her peers (unless the child has a natural aptitude for math which may give him/her social opportunities among other children who are proficient in math).

More About Place Value (Advanced)

Each place has a value 10 times more than the column to its right.
    This means that as you **MOVE TO THE LEFT IN PLACE VALUE,**
    the **NUMBERS GET BIGGER.**
    As you **MOVE TO THE LEFT OF THE DECIMAL POINT,**
    the **NUMBERS GET LARGER.**

When you look at a number, you can tell what each digit means by looking at the digit's place value.
The number 2 has one digit. The 2 is in the ones place. This means that there are 2 groups of 1 in the number 2.

The number 10 has two digits. The 1 is in the tens place. The 0 is in the ones place. This means that there is 1 group of 10, but 0 or no groups of 1.
It means the same thing as 10 + 0 (zero) or 10.

The number 238 has three digits. The 2 is in the hundreds place. The 3 is in the tens place. The 8 is in the ones place.
This means that there are 2 groups of 100, 3 groups of 10, and 8 groups of 1.
It means the same thing as 200 + 30 + 8 or 238.

WHEN YOU READ A NUMBER, ALWAYS START WITH THE FIRST DIGIT ON THE LEFT - THE DIGIT IN THE HIGHEST PLACE VALUE.

Then, think about the place value of the first digit.
To read the number 348, you start with the 3.
You know that the 3 is in the hundreds place, so you say, "Three hundred forty-eight."

KNOWING ABOUT PLACE VALUE IS IMPORTANT.
KNOWING ABOUT PLACE VALUE TEACHES YOU ABOUT NUMBERS.

Place Value Continued (Advanced)

The visual representation of the advanced place value script should be introduced at the same time as the script since it relates directly to what is explained in the script.

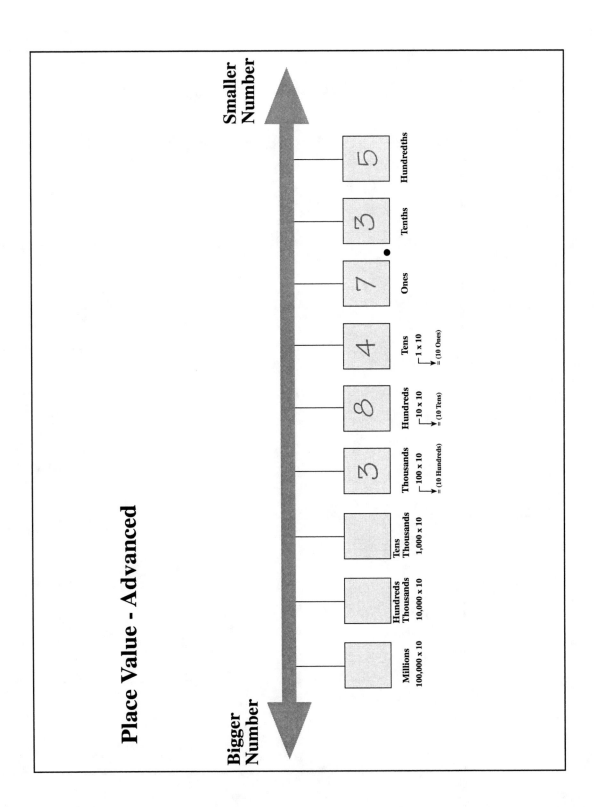

Understanding Place Value

The Understanding Place Value exercise reinforces what has been learned in the Place Value script. The goal is for the child to understand what the number means to prevent him/her from falling behind in math due to difficulty in grasping language based math concepts.

Understanding Place Value

Look at each number. Tell how many digits it has. Then tell what each digit means.

Number	How many digits	What each digit means
6, 492	4	The 6 means 6 one thousands
		The 4 means 4 one hundreds
		The 9 means 9 tens
		The 2 means 2 ones
5,998	4	The 5 means 5 one thousands
		The 9 means 9 one hundreds
		The 9 means 9 tens
		The 8 means 8 ones

How To Teach Comparative Words

There are two exercises designed to teach comparative words. The first exercise, Using Comparatives, has the child find opposite examples of objects based on the type of comparison that the therapist has specified. This is a very versatile exercise since a large number of comparative concepts can be learned by using the template provided. The second Using Comparatives sheet is designed to teach comparatives that have more than two relative states e.g. small, smaller, smallest, or hot, hotter, hottest. This sheet lends itself to be used with three dimensional objects when possible. In both comparative exercises, the therapist should prompt the child through the sheet until s/he understands the structure. Once the child understands what is required of him/her, the child should be able to concentrate on learning the relative concepts.

Note: We have provided a list of examples of relative (comparative) concepts that should be taught. This list is by no means exhaustive. In fact, the child will come across comparative concepts which can be explained throughout his/her childhood using the following drills.

Why Teach Comparative Words

Comparative words are important to teach because they are common in both stories and factual text. In addition, arithmetic requires the understanding of comparatives words. Furthermore, comparative words are related to sequencing which is an important competence to work towards.

Comparative Words To Be Taught

Throughout the child's life, s/he is going to come across the following list of comparison categorizes and words. It is important that these concepts be taught. Some of the concepts can be taught using the number sequencing exercises, others need to be taught using the following Comparison exercises.

Measurement/Size

big/bigger/biggest
large/larger/largest

small/smaller/smallest
little/littler/littlest
tiny/tinier/tiniest

tall/taller/tallest
short/shorter/shortest
long/longer/longest

thin/thinner/thinnest
skinny/skinnier/skinniest

fat/fatter/fattest
wide/wider/widest

Quantity/Money

many/more/most
less/least/fewest

expensive/more expensive/
most expensive
cheap/cheaper/cheapest

Weight

heavy/heavier/heaviest
light/lighter/lightest

Temperature

hot/hotter/hottest
cold/colder/coldest

Age

old/older/oldest
young/younger/youngest

Using Comparatives - Sheet 1

This exercise has the child compare relative size by using material that the child is familiar with, in this case animal size. When preparing this sheet, the therapist should draw lines from one adjective to another, making sure that there are obvious differences in what is being compared.

Using Comparatives - Sheet 1

Look at the comparative adjectives on the line. Use one of the comparative words to make a sentence about the two word pairs.

Comparatives: _bigger/smaller_

elephant

lion ———→snake

lizard   turtle

ant   zebra

whale

An elephant is bigger than an ant.

A lizard is smaller than a zebra.

A turtle is smaller than a whale.

A lion is bigger than a snake.

Using Comparatives - Sheet 2

This exercise has the child compare relative size using three objects. This is a much more difficult exercise than the Using Comparatives - Sheet 1 because the child must 1) order three objects, and 2) generate original ideas about the relationship of the objects to other items. The therapist writes the questions and the child answers orally.

Using Comparatives - Sheet 2

Put the small square things under the correct box.

Three Sample Objects:

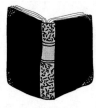

small	smaller	smallest
book	ring bot	dice

Which is _the smallest?_
Which is _the biggest?_
Is the dice bigger than the book?
Is the ring box bigger than the dice?

Think of something that is _smaller than the dice._

Think of something that is _bigger than the book._

Put the 3 things in order from _small to smallest._

1. _book_
2. _ring bot_
3. _dice_

How To Teach Calendar

Children with pervasive developmental disorders should be exposed to the calendar every therapy session for many years. This is a concept that the child masters after a substantial amount of time. Some children take years to master the calendar while others never completely understand the calendar due to the significant role of sequencing which is intrinsic to calendar skills.

1. The child must be taught the concept of days, weeks, months and years. The way to teach these concepts is outlined in the section on TIME. Once the child has been introduced to the relationship between days, weeks, months, and years (i.e. that there are 7 days in a week, 28-31 days in a month, 4 -5 weeks in a month, 12 months in a year, 365 days in a year) then the therapist can proceed to Step 2. At this point, the child needs to work on Steps 1 and 2 at the same time until the child masters Step 1.

2. The Monthly Calendar is introduced. First, the therapist should use the template to ACCURATELY reproduce the current month. Next, the child should be asked a variety of questions from the Calendar Script and be given the opportunity to use the Monthly Calendar to count and thereby answer the questions from the script.

3. Once the child is able to answer the questions in the Calendar Script, s/he should be given the opportunity to complete the Monthly Calendar Fill-In which has been prepared by the therapist before hand. The child should be helped to complete the Monthly Calendar Fill-In until s/he understands the questions. At this point, the therapist should fade into the background and the child should complete this sheet by him/herself.

4. The next step is to teach the child "Today", "Yesterday" and "Tomorrow". This is taught by using today as a reference. The child must answer the question by writing in the calender. For example, the therapist says, "Today is here" (and points to the box). Then she says, "Yesterday I went to the store" and the child must write "Store" in the appropriate box. Once the child can do this quite well, the therapist should teach "Last Friday" and "Next Tuesday" using the same technique. "Last" and "Next", as they relate to calendar, are very difficult to teach.

5. Finally, the "Using the Correct Tense" sheet should be introduced using the calendar so that the child learns the relationship between Past, Present and Future and Yesterday, Today, Tomorrow. The therapist says, "Tomorrow, I will go swimming." Then the therapist says, "Tell me what I will do". The child must say, "Tomorrow, you will go swimming." Once the child can do this, the "Verb Tense" sheet can be used. This is an exceptionally difficult task and may take a long time for even the brightest child to master.

Why Teach Calendar?

The ability to use a calendar is one of those skills that the child needs in order to understand verb tense. In addition, calendar is taught in kindergarten and first grade and is a concept that is constantly used in daily life. Therefore, it is important to teach calendar skills. Many parents may think that their child has calendar skills because the child can recite the days of the week or months of the year. A good memory, unfortunately, does not guarantee that the child understands what s/he has memorized and the wise parent will do these drills until the child can answer all the questions asked, including questions that concern tense. In this way, the child will truly learn tense and sequence.

Monthly Calendar

This calendar (which should be filled out every month) is designed to accompany the calendar script. It is also a good idea to have a large calendar upon which the child can write significant events. To teach verb tense, the child can be asked about what s/he did yesterday, what she is doing today, and what she is going to do tomorrow.

Month:_____

Sun.	Mon.	Tue.	Wed.	Th.	Fri.	Sat.

Calendar Script

This script should be done with the child every day for each month until the child can easily answer all the questions. The child should also be able to 1) name the date s/he was born on, 2) locate it on the calendar, 3) be able to ask when a family member's birthday is, and write it on his/her calendar. The child should master this drill relatively quickly since it relies on rote memorization. Once the child can answers all the questions by looking at the script and calendar, it is important to remove the script. The goal of this exercise is for the child to listen to the question, and locate the answer on the calendar, without using the script as a visual prompt.

Calendar Script

Each month the child should be asked the following questions:

How many days are in _September_ ?

What month comes before _September_ ?

What month comes after _September_ ?

How many _Mon_ days are in _September_ ? (vary this)

Are there more _Mon_ days than _Fri_ days in _September_ ? (vary this)

What day of the week is the _first_ of _September_ ? (vary this)

What day is the first day of _September_ on?

What day is the last day of _September_ on?

General questions the child should be able to answer (after being worked with):

How many days are in a week?

How many months are in a year?

Name the months in order.

After listing the months, be able to name the ordinal position of a specific month.

Name the seasons.

When give a month, be able to tell the season it is in.

Know what month the following holidays are in (customize to each child in terms of religious holidays):

New Year's Day   Independence Day
Valentine's Day   Labor Day
St. Patrick's Day   Halloween
Easter   Thanksgiving
Memorial Day   Christmas

Monthly Calendar Fill-In

At the beginning of every month, the child should complete this sheet using a calendar to refer to. This will help maintain the calendar skills learned from the calendar script and calendar drills. Eventually, the child should be able to know, without looking at a calendar, the month before and the month after the current month. Other than that the child SHOULD NOT be encouraged to memorize mundane calendar facts (e.g. how many Mondays there are in August).

Monthly Calendar Fill-In

Read each sentence. Fill in the correct answer.

There are _31_ **days in** _August_ .

The first day of _August_ **is on a** _Mon_ **day.**

The last day of _August_ **is on a** _Wednes_ **day.**

The _16th_ **of** _August_ **is on a** _Tues_ **day.**

The _21st_ **of** _August_ **is on a** _Sun_ **day.**

There are _four_ _Fri_ **days in** _August_ .

There are _five_ _Tues_ **days in** _August_ .

July **is the month before** _August_ .

September **is the month after** _August_ .

Using The Correct Verb Tense

This exercise works on the child's verb tenses. The sheet should be customized to the child in order for the verb tenses to have meaning. If the child is supposed to conjugate a verb with "Yesterday", the therapist must use a verb that reflects what the child did yesterday. The more the therapist can relate the child's experience with the language being taught, the more sense that concept will make to the child.

Note: The therapist should set up the sheet to reflect the concepts that the child is working on at the moment. Once the child has learned past, present and future and is fairly good at conjugating verb tenses, then the concepts should be mixed (such as they are in this sheet).

Using The Correct Verb Tense

Read each sentence. Circle the correct verb tense.

Tomorrow I will ((go) , went) to school.

I already ((ate) , eat) breakfast.

I already (do , (did)) my homework.

Yesterday I (will go , (went)) on a bike ride.

Today I am (took , (taking)) a bath.

Complete each sentence (let the child use his personal calendar initially).

Tomorrow I will go to the park.

I already ate my dinner.

Cards For Teaching Calendar

These are reproducible calendar cards to be used as explained on the previous page. They can be photocopied onto card stock to ensure their durability.

cut ✂

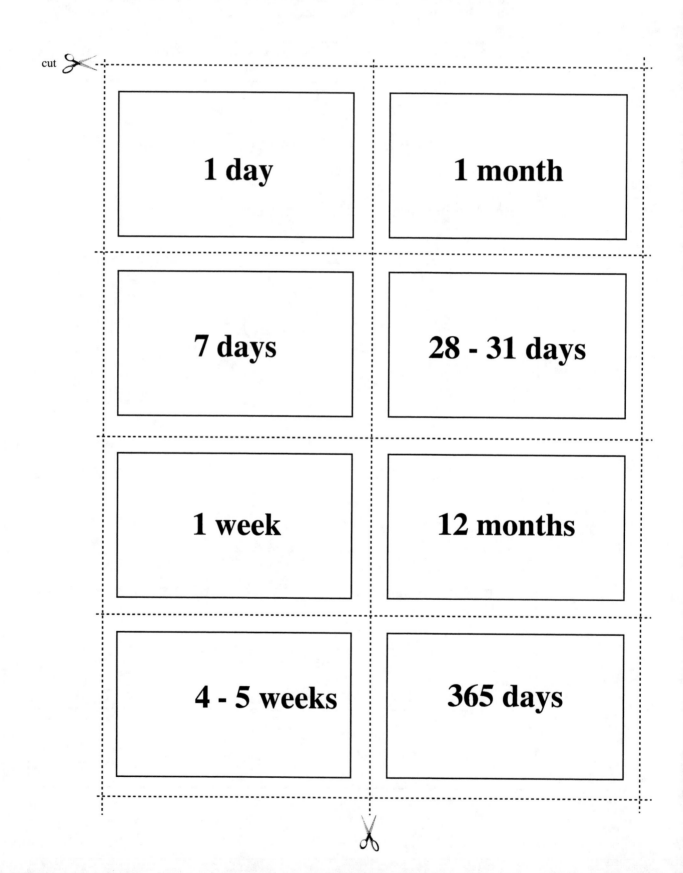

1 day	**1 month**
7 days	**28 - 31 days**
1 week	**12 months**
4 - 5 weeks	**365 days**

Cards For Teaching Calendar

These are reproducible calendar cards to be used as explained on the previous pages. They can be photocopied onto card stock to ensure their durability.

1 year	**April**
January	**May**
February	**June**
March	**July**

Cards For Teaching Calendar

These are reproducible calendar cards to be used as explained on the previous pages. They can be photocopied onto card stock to ensure their durability.

August	**December**
September	**Monday**
October	**Tuesday**
November	**Wednesday**

Cards For Teaching Calendar

These are reproducible calendar cards to be used as explained on the previous pages. They can be photocopied onto card stock to ensure their durability.

cut ✂

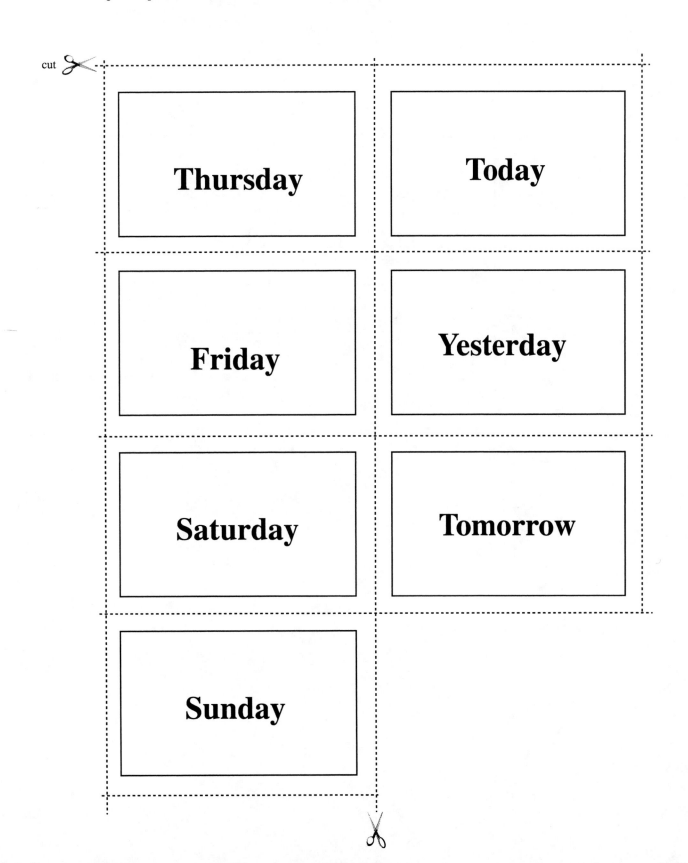

Thursday	Today
Friday	Yesterday
Saturday	Tomorrow
Sunday	

Cards For Teaching Calendar

These are reproducible calendar cards to be used as explained on the previous pages. They can be photocopied onto card stock to ensure their durability.

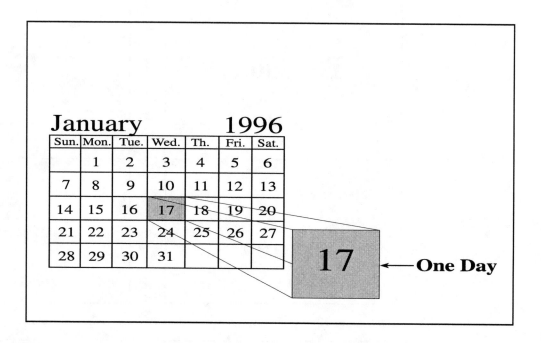

Cards For Teaching Calendar

These are reproducible calendar cards to be used as explained on the previous pages. They can be photocopied onto card stock to ensure their durability.

January 1996

Sun.	Mon.	Tue.	Wed.	Th.	Fri.	Sat.
	1	2	3	4	5	6
7	8	9	10	11	12	13
14	15	16	17	18	19	20
21	22	23	24	25	26	27
28	29	30	31			

← **One Week**

January 1996

Sun.	Mon.	Tue.	Wed.	Th.	Fri.	Sat.
	1	2	3	4	5	6
7	8	9	10	11	12	13
14	15	16	17	18	19	20
21	22	23	24	25	26	27
28	29	30	31			

One Month

Cards For Teaching Calendar

These are reproducible calendar cards to be used as explained on the previous pages. They can be photocopied onto card stock to ensure their durability.

One Year - 1996

1996

January

Sun.	Mon.	Tue.	Wed.	Th.	Fri.	Sat.
	1	2	3	4	5	6
7	8	9	10	11	12	13
14	15	16	17	18	19	20
21	22	23	24	25	26	27
28	29	30	31			

February

Sun.	Mon.	Tue.	Wed.	Th.	Fri.	Sat.
				1	2	3
4	5	6	7	8	9	10
11	12	13	14	15	16	17
18	19	20	21	22	23	24
25	26	27	28	29	30	31

March

Sun.	Mon.	Tue.	Wed.	Th.	Fri.	Sat.
					1	2
3	4	5	6	7	8	9
10	11	12	13	14	15	16
17	18	19	20	21	22	23
24 / 31	25	26	27	28	29	30

April

Sun.	Mon.	Tue.	Wed.	Th.	Fri.	Sat.
	1	2	3	4	5	6
7	8	9	10	11	12	13
14	15	16	17	18	19	20
21	22	23	24	25	26	27
28	29	30				

May

Sun.	Mon.	Tue.	Wed.	Th.	Fri.	Sat.
			1	2	3	4
5	6	7	8	9	10	11
12	13	14	15	16	17	18
19	20	21	22	23	24	25
26	27	28	29	30	31	

June

Sun.	Mon.	Tue.	Wed.	Th.	Fri.	Sat.
						1
2	3	4	5	6	7	8
9	10	11	12	13	14	15
16	17	18	19	20	21	22
23 / 30	24	25	26	27	28	29

July

Sun.	Mon.	Tue.	Wed.	Th.	Fri.	Sat.
	1	2	3	4	5	6
7	8	9	10	11	12	13
14	15	16	17	18	19	20
21	22	23	24	25	26	27
28	29	30	31			

August

Sun.	Mon.	Tue.	Wed.	Th.	Fri.	Sat.
				1	2	3
4	5	6	7	8	9	10
11	12	13	14	15	16	17
18	19	20	21	22	23	24
25	26	27	28	29	30	31

September

Sun.	Mon.	Tue.	Wed.	Th.	Fri.	Sat.
1	2	3	4	5	6	7
8	9	10	11	12	13	14
15	16	17	18	19	20	21
22	23	24	25	26	27	28
29	30	31				

October

Sun.	Mon.	Tue.	Wed.	Th.	Fri.	Sat.
		1	2	3	4	5
6	7	8	9	10	11	12
13	14	15	16	17	18	19
20	21	22	23	24	25	26
27	28	29	30	31		

November

Sun.	Mon.	Tue.	Wed.	Th.	Fri.	Sat.
					1	2
3	4	5	6	7	8	9
10	11	12	13	14	15	16
17	18	19	20	21	22	23
24	25	26	27	28	29	30

December

Sun.	Mon.	Tue.	Wed.	Th.	Fri.	Sat.
1	2	3	4	5	6	7
8	9	10	11	12	13	14
15	16	17	18	19	20	21
22	23	24	25	26	27	28
29	30	31				

How to Teach Sequencing A Day

Sequencing the child's day must be taught incrementally. Each step should be mastered before moving on to the next step:

Step 1: Ordering the Cards
The first step is to teach the child the sequence of the day using a minimal number of cards i.e. morning; afternoon; night. Once the child understands this, then the full number of cards that relate to parts of day can be introduced i.e. early morning, morning, noon, afternoon, evening, night, midnight.

Next, the child should be able to order "Yesterday", "Today" and "Tomorrow" in the correct order. The child should know this from calendar skills taught before "Sequencing A Day".

Step 2: Before - After
Once the child can order the cards, then s/he should be taught to order them from "Before" to "After", and "After" to "Before".

Step 3: Earlier - Later
The concept of earlier and later should be introduced and the child should be able to order the cards from "Earlier" to "Later", and "Later" to "Earlier".

Step 4: Pairing Events to Parts of Day
Once the child understands the sequence of the parts of the day, then the events that take place in that part of the day should be paired. For example, "morning" should be paired with "eat breakfast", "Eat lunch" should be paired with "Noon". All the events that always take place at a certain time of day should be used and the cards should be customized to the particular child (if the child does not take piano, DO NOT use the "Go to Piano" card). Over time, the parts of the day should take on some relevance to the child's life and s/he should come to understand the concept of parts of the day.

Why Teach Sequencing of Day?

Sequencing is a major deficit of the majority of children with developmental disorders. Teaching sequencing by using the child's day helps make sequencing relevant to the child. In this way, the child is more likely to grasp the concept of sequencing. Once the child understands sequencing, concepts of calendar, and time become easier to grasp.

Cards To Teach Sequencing of Day

These are reproducible sequencing cards to be used as explained on the previous page. They can be photocopied onto card stock to ensure their durability.

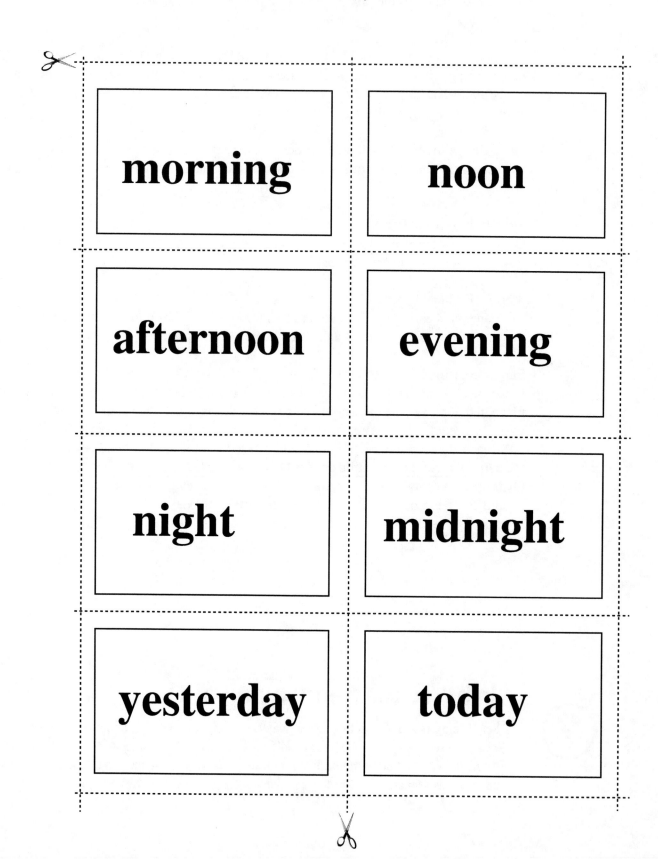

morning	**noon**
afternoon	**evening**
night	**midnight**
yesterday	**today**

Cards To Teach Sequencing of Day

These are reproducible sequencing cards to be used as explained on the previous page. They can be photocopied onto card stock to ensure their durability.

tomorrow	**early morning**
Before	**After**
Earlier	**Later**
go to Grandma's	**go to Gymnastics**

Cards To Teach Sequencing of Day

These are reproducible sequencing cards to be used as explained on the previous page. They can be photocopied onto card stock to ensure their durability.

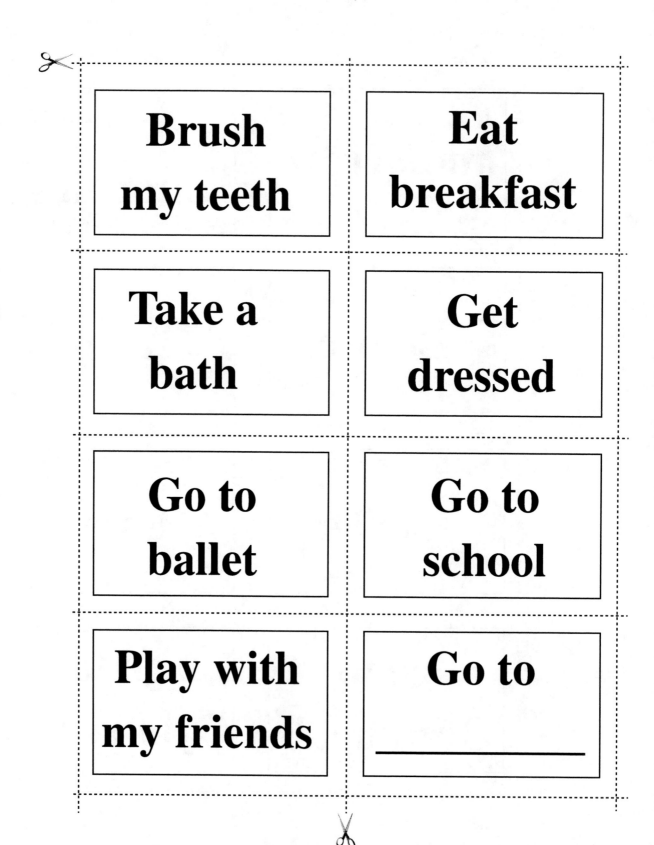

Brush my teeth	Eat breakfast
Take a bath	Get dressed
Go to ballet	Go to school
Play with my friends	Go to _____

Cards To Teach Sequencing of Day

These are reproducible sequencing cards to be used as explained on the previous page. They can be photocopied onto card stock to ensure their durability.

Eat Lunch	**Go swimming**
Do homework	**Wake up**
Go to bed	**Put on pyjamas**
Eat dinner	**Go to piano lessons**

What Happens?

This exercise has the child match a period of time with an activity that the child does at that time. Each sheet needs to be customized to the specific child. For example, if the child goes to gymnastics on Saturday morning, the therapist should use Saturday morning as one of the periods of time to describe the event. The more meaningful the activities and the more varied the times, the greater likelihood that the child will understand this concept.

What Happens?

Look at each period of time and answer the question.

What <u>is something you do</u> ?   *Event*

on Saturday	go to Ballet class
on Monday	go to school
in the morning	eat breakfast
in the evening	eat dinner
on Friday	work with Sandy

When <u>do you go to school</u> ?   <u>in the morning</u>

When <u>do you go to</u> ?   <u>in the afternoon</u>
<u>swimming lessons</u>

AM Or PM Time

This exercise has the child match an activity to the A.M. or P.M. This is a much harder exercise than the previous one because the concept of A.M. and P.M. is abstract. Before this exercise is introduced, the child must be shown on a blackboard or piece of paper that A.M. refers to all time from 12:00 in the early morning to 11:59 in the late morning, and that P.M. refers to all time from 12:00 noon (lunchtime) to 11:59 at night. Although this is a Sequencing A Day exercise, it should not be introduced until the child is learning "Time".

AM Or PM Time

Look at each event or thing that happens.
Tell whether the event happens in the A.M. or P.M.

Event	A.M. or P.M.?
go to Ballet class	a.m.
go to school	a.m.
eat breakfast	a.m.
eat dinner	p.m.
work with Sandy	p.m.

What is something you might do during A.M. hours?

wake up, go to school, have recess, eat breakfast, get dressed

What is something you might do during P.M. hours?

do homework, eat dinner, work with Sandy, watch T.V. with Dad

How To Teach Time

Teaching time is a very difficult skill. We are not talking about the child's ability to tell time; we are referring to the child's ability to grasp the concept of time. The concept of time is related to the ability to sequence which is a weak spot for the majority of children with developmental disorders. We provide several different ways to target this deficit: STEP 1, the therapist reads the Time Script and looks at the Time Line with the child. The therapist should read one line, and the child should read the other (if the child is a pre-reader, introduction of this skill is premature, and time should not be a priority). The Time Script should be read once each therapy session for many therapy sessions (20 or 30 sessions). Once the child knows this script well, then the therapist can introduce Step Two. At this point, the child is expected to know the script well, but not yet understand the concept of time.

STEP 2, read the Time Teaching Hierarchy which follows the Time Script and introduce the card drills, following the order closely.

STEP 3, have the child work on the following drills:
> When Phrase Drill
> Sequences The Child Should Learn
> Sequencing A Day (using the cards)
> Sequencing Parts Of The Day (with the cards)
> What Happens?
> AM Or PM Time?

Why Teach Time?

The concept of time is important because it is another channel to use to target the problem of sequencing (which is a requisite skill for comprehending most language, whether written, or spoken). Aside from the obvious role of time in modern society, time also orders experiences since most of what we do is naturally sequenced. For example, when eating in a restaurant, first, people are seated, then, they eat, and last, they pay. These activities can be measured in units of time. In this way, the concept of time plays an implicit, as well as explicit, role.

Time

When the child has mastered sequencing with numbers and some calendar skills, s/he is ready to learn about time. (Money can be introduced before or after but not at the same time). This script is designed to be read with the child, emphasizing the words in bold as they are read. The script can also be read by the child and therapist alternating lines. The script should be in much larger format (on a full sheet of paper) to make it easy to read. Once the script is read, the visual representation which follows should be explained by the therapist. This must be done daily in order for the child to learn the script. Once the child understands the script, then the questions in the script should be asked verbally, without using the script.

Time

TIME tells us **HOW LONG** it takes for something to happen.

It takes about 1 hour to bake a cake. 1 hour is **HOW LONG** it

takes to bake a cake.

TIME tells us **WHEN TO DO SOMETHING**.

School starts at 8:30 in the morning. 8:30 in the morning is

WHEN you go to school.

TIME tells us **WHEN SOMETHING WILL HAPPEN.**

Christmas is on December 25. December 25 is the day **WHEN**

Christmas is celebrated.

WATCHES and **CLOCKS** tell us about **TIME** in seconds, minutes,

and hours.

CALENDARS tell us about **TIME** in **days, weeks, and months**.

TIME can be **short** or **long.**

One second is a **short time.**

One year is a **long time.**

Time Line

This visual representation of time should be introduced to the child after s/he has worked on the Time Script. These two tools complement each other and should always be presented together.

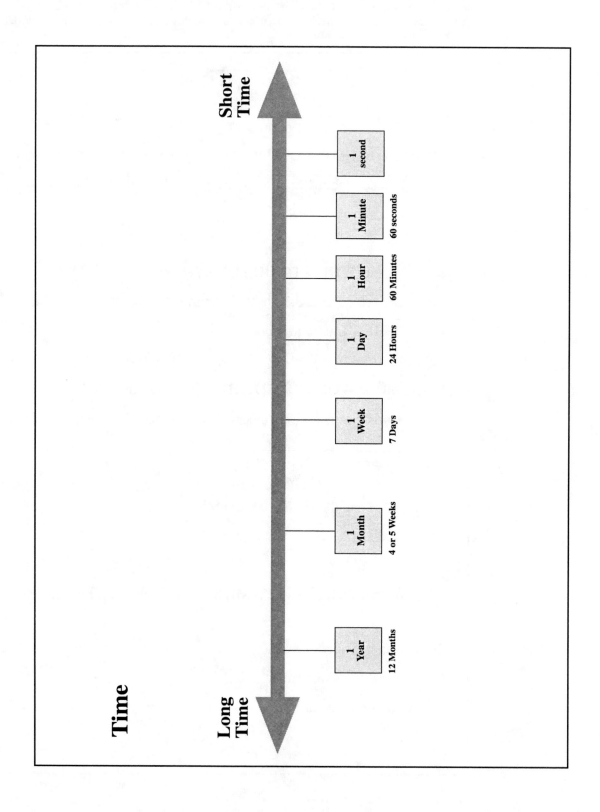

Time Teaching Hierarchy

The Time Teaching Hierarchy introduces the child to time through sequencing units of time (e.g. 1 hour, 1 minute, 1 second). As the child learns to sequence time, s/he needs to get a "feel" for how long a second, a minute, and an hour actually is. This requires showing the child how long familiar daily activities take. As the child does short activities (such as brushing teeth, or tying shoes), the therapist should use a stopwatch to visually show the child how long the activity takes. Acquiring a sense of time takes much experience; as the child is exposed to this technique through measuring and sequencing time units, the concept of time will become clearer.

Time should be taught in the following order using the time cards provided in <u>Teach Me Language</u>:

1. Sequencing - More Time/Less Time, and Shorter Amount of Time/Longer Amount of Time.

In this exercise, the therapist must organize the time cards into four sets:
      (1) 1 second, 1 minute, 1 hour
      (2) 1 day, 1 week, 1 month, 1 year
      (3) more time, less time
      (4) longer amount of time, shorter amount of time

The therapist uses Set 1 and Set 3 to begin. She lays them out so that at one end of the table is the "more time" card, and at the other is the "less time" card. The therapist shows the child how to order 1 second, 1 minute, and 1 hour relative to the "more time" and "less time" cards. Next, the therapist should reverse the position of the "more time" and "less time" cards and have the child sequence the cards again. Then the therapist should put the "more time" card at the top of the table, and the "less time" card at the bottom of the table and have the child do the sequence again. Finally, the therapist should switch the "more time" and "less time" cards and have the child do the sequence one more time. Once the child can do this well, then the therapist should introduce Set 4, showing the child that "more time" equals "longer amount of time", and "less time" equals "shorter amount of time". The therapist should have the child order the same time cards using Set 4 cards. Once the child can order these cards easily, the same exercise should be done with Set 2. When the child can easily order Set 2, than Set 1 and Set 2 should be combined and the child should be asked to order the 7 time cards using Sets 3 and 4 interchangeably.

The child should learn this skill relatively quickly (over the span of a few therapy sessions). This chapter provides cards to visually represent the units of time which should be used initially. The use of a visual representation for each time unit may not seem necessary, since the child may be able to sequence the units using word cards only; however, it is very important the child understand "more" time, and "less" time. The visual time cards help with this concept and are an efficient way to represent time. Once the child can sequence the cards as directed above, the "Sequencing Time" drill sheet should be used to develop and maintain this skill.

2. Comparing - More Time/Less Time, and Shorter Amount of Time/Longer Amount of Time.

In this exercise, the therapist takes the time cards that have been sequenced by the child, and has the child compare two units of time (1 hour versus 1 second, 1 month versus 1 year, etc.) and identify the following:

      a. which unit of time takes "more time"
      b. which unit of time takes "less time"
      c. which unit of time takes a "longer amount of time"
      d. which unit of time takes a "shorter amount of time"

This is an example of how the exercise would sound:
Therapist: "What takes more time, 1 hour or 1 minute?"
Child: "1 hour."
Therapist: "What takes less time, 1 hour or 1 minute?"
Child: "1 minute."
Therapist: "What takes a longer amount of time, 1 hour or 1 minute?"
Child: "1 hour."
Therapist: "What takes a shorter amount of time, 1 hour or 1 minute?"
Child: "1 minute."

Initially, the therapist should set up the exercise with the time cards in front of the child in sequence. Then the therapist must take two of the cards to compare, pulling them out of the sequence. Once the child can compare time cards using a variety of two card combinations, the child should be asked to compare the two cards without the sequenced cards in view. The therapist should ask, "What takes more/less time? A second or a minute", etc. This should be done with all the possible combinations of two cards. Eventually, the two cards being compared should be removed entirely, and the child should be able to answer the same questions when asked orally. Once the child can complete this exercise without the cards, the "Comparing Time" drill sheet can be used to practise this skill.

3. Tell time accurately

It is important that the child be able to tell time. If the child has not learned to tell time, this should be taught before continuing according to the time hierarchy. The child should know what "half past/to the hour" and "quarter past/to the hour" means. This can be taught using several different methods. We recommend using "Discrete Trial Training" to tell time. The ME book and Behavioral Intervention for Children With Autism (both cited in Chapter 1) go into great detail regarding this technique.

4. Equivalencies - Same and Different with Units of Time

This step teaches the child that the same amount of time can be represented in different ways. Specifically, the child needs to know that 1 minute is the same as 60 seconds, 1 hour is the same as 60 minutes, 1 day is the same as 24 hours, 1 week is the same as 7 days, 4 weeks is the same as 28 - 31 days or 1 month, and 1 year is the same as 12 months or 365 days. In short, the child needs to be taught that each larger unit of time can be equally represented by using smaller units of time. The cards for this drill can be found in the Calendar section and Time section of this chapter.

The therapist begins this exercise by having the child match two cards that represent the equivalent amount of time. For example, the therapist would put out the "1 year" card and the "1 month" card. Then she would give the child the "365 days" card and have the child match it to the "1 year" card. The matching should be done with all the possible combinations. Once the child can match these equivalent time units, the child should be asked questions about all the equivalent time units s/he has matched. Examples of questions include, "How many hours are in a day?", and "How many days are in a year?" The child should be able to answer correctly when asked first answering while matching the cards, and then without the cards in view. In addition, the child should be able to sequence these time units. Sequencing the time units should not be difficult for the child if the sequencing time units have already been taught (as is recommended). The child should learn to sequence using groups of equivalent cards interchangeably if the therapist spent enough time sequencing with the cards the Sequencing Coins and Bills section above. If the child does have difficulty, it is a good idea to refresh the child's skills by returning to the section on sequencing. Once the child can sequence equivalent units interchangeably using the cards, the therapist can introduce the "Time Equivalents" drill sheet.

5. Comparing - More Time/Same Amount of Time/Less Time, and Shorter Amount of Time/Same Amount of Time/Longer Amount of Time.

This exercise is similar to the comparison exercise in Step 2; however, in this exercise the child must be able to identify "Same Amount of Time" as well. A large variety of equivalent times should be used. Examples include 2 weeks versus 14 days; 5 months versus 10 weeks, 2 months versus 8 weeks, 48 hours versus 2 days. Equivalencies which the child will never encounter (such as 2 years versus 104 weeks) should not be taught. At this stage, the goal is to have the child understand how to use his/her knowledge about equivalent amounts of time.

First, the therapist has the child sequence the time cards. Then she should have the child compare two units of time (1 hour versus 1 minute, 1 day versus 24 hours, 2 weeks versus 1 month, etc.). The child should be asked to identify:
> a. which unit of time takes more time
> Therapist: "What takes more time, (1 hour) or (1 day)?"
> b. which unit of time takes less time
> Therapist: "What takes less time, (1 hour) or (1 day)?"
> c. which unit of time takes a longer amount of time
> Therapist: "What takes a longer amount of time, (1 hour) or (1 day)?"
> d. which unit of time takes a shorter amount of time
> Therapist: "What takes a shorter amount of time, (1 hour) or (1 day)?"
> e. which units of time takes the same amount of time
> Therapist: "What takes the same amount of time, (1 hour), (1 day), (24 hours)?"

Note: While this concept is being taught in therapy, time must relate to the child's daily life. Therefore, adults should point out to the child how much time a particular activity takes (e.g. baking a cake, or watching a television program).

Once the child has completed all the above steps, the therapist can introduce the "Time Questions" sheet. This sheet should be used until the child can easily answer all the questions and <u>understands</u> the relative time questions (the first 5 questions on the "Time Questions" sheet).

Sequencing Time

In this exercise, the child sequences time according to the instructions at the top of the sheet which are customized by the therapist based on the Teaching Time Hierarchy. The example uses "shorter to longer" time amounts. The child should also sequence "longer to shorter", "less time" to "more time", and "more time" to "less time".

Sequencing Time

Put the time amounts in order from: _shortest amount of time to longest amount of time_

1 day, 1 minute, 1 second | second | minute | day

1 week, 1 year, 1 minute | minute | week | year

1 month, 1 week, 1 year | week | month | year

1 minute, 1 year, 1 second | second | minute | year

Comparing Time

In this exercise the child compares time by its relative length. This should be relatively easy for the child if s/he has mastered time using the time cards. If this drill is difficult, the therapist should return to the cards for a refresher session.

Comparing Time

Look at each amount of time.
Circle the amount that:

is shorter   (1 day)   1 year   1 week

is longer   1 hour   week   (1 minute)

is longer   (1 month)   1 week   1 minute

is shorter   (1 second)   1 year   1 day

Time Equivalents

In this exercise the child identifies the amount of time that is equivalent to the amount of time on the left-hand side of the page. This drill should be relatively easy for the child if s/he has learned time from the cards. If the child has difficulty completing this drill, the therapist should return to the cards until the child has mastered time using the time cards.

Time Equivalents

Look at each amount of time.
Circle the amount or amounts of time that are the same.

1 minute   28-31 days   1 week   (60 seconds)

1 week   60 minutes   (7 days)   3 months

1 month   12 hours   (4-5 weeks)   (28-31 days)

1 hour   60 days   (60 minutes)   60 seconds

Time Questions

This exercise has the child think about the concept of time by comparing amounts of time. The exercise also helps maintain what the child has learned about time from the preceding exercises. These questions are asked orally to the child. The question sheet should be customized to the specific child, where appropriate.

Time Questions

Which takes longer, brushing your teeth or taking a bath? ___taking a bath___

Which takes less time, typing your shoes or watching the Jungle Book? ___tying shoes___

Which takes longer, baking a cake or eating a bowl or cereal? ___baking a cake___

Which takes less time, doing your homework, or brushing your hair? ___brushing___

Which is the most amount of time - 24 hours or 2 days? ___2 days___

How many days are in a week? ___7 days___

How many hours in a day? ___24 hours___

How many seconds in a minute? ___60 seconds___

How many months in a year? ___12 months___

How many days in a month? ___28-31 days___

What happens at school at 10 o'clock? ___recess___

What happens at around 8:30? ___school begins___

What time is morning recess? ___10:00___

What time does school start? ___8:30___

When is lunch? ___12:00___

What do you do at about 10:30? ___reading with Mrs. Smith___

How To Do The When Phrase Drill

Using the sheet provided, the therapist should write two times of day e.g. in the morning, at night. Then the therapist should say, "Tell me three things you do in the morning." If the child does not understand, then the therapist should prompt the child with the first answer e.g. "I eat breakfast." Eventually, the child will come to understand what IN THE MORNING means. Once the child has completed the form (with the therapist's help), then the therapist should ask the question again and the child should use the form to answer. Then, the therapist should ask the child again, but this time the therapist must remove the sheet. Once the child understands the exercise, then the therapist should ask the child a when question. For example, the therapist could ask, "When do you eat breakfast?" The child will soon understand that "When" questions refer to parts of the day (in their many forms).

The therapist should begin by using the simplest parts of the day (morning, afternoon, night). Once the child understands these basic times, then the therapist should add harder concepts (evening, lunch, dinner). Eventually more abstract types of WHEN should be used (in the summer, at a birthday party, at school, **during** recess, **after** lunch, **before** school). These variations may take some time for the child to master. Eventually, the child should come to understand the concept of when.

Why Do the When Phrase Drill?

Often children with language delays have a difficulty with time concepts. Although they may learn to tell time relatively easily, the abstract notion of time is still difficult for them. The WHEN drill has the child pair activities that s/he does with WHEN s/he does them. The hope is that the child will, over time, come to understand that WHEN refers to time. Once the child understands this concept, the next steps are to work on the child answering and asking WHEN questions.

When Phrases

This exercise has the child list activities that s/he does at certain times of the day. Other times of the day that can be used in the exercise are: at breakfast, at recess, at lunch, at dinner, in the evening, after school, on Saturday (any day of the week), before school, before bedtime, during recess, etc.

When Phrases

Write down 3 things that you do:

__in the morning__   ___at night___

1. _eat breakfast_   1. ___eat dinner___

2. _brush my teeth_   2. __practise piano__

3. _get dressed_   3. __put pyjamas on__

Cards For Teaching Time

These are reproducible time cards to be used as explained in the Time Hierarchy on the previous pages. These cards can be photocopied onto card stock to ensure their durability.

1 second	**60 minutes**
1 minute	**24 hours**
1 hour	**1 day**
60 seconds	

Cards For Teaching Time

These are reproducible time cards to be used according to the Time Hierarchy described earlier. These cards can be photocopied onto card stock to ensure their durability.

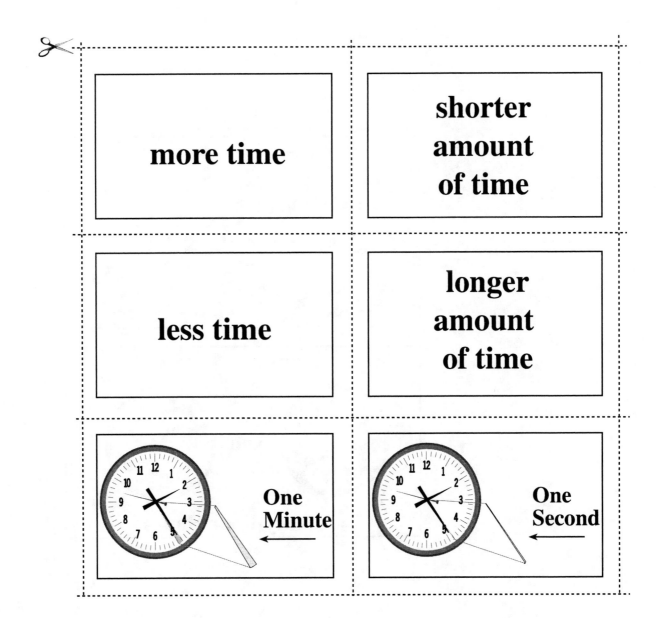

more time	shorter amount of time
less time	longer amount of time
One Minute	One Second

Cards For Teaching Time

These are reproducible time cards to be used as described in the Time Hierarchy on the preceding pages. These cards can be photocopied onto card stock to ensure their durability.

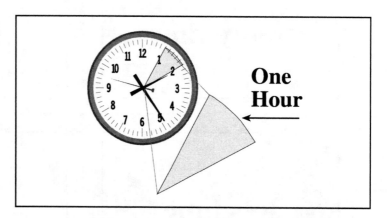

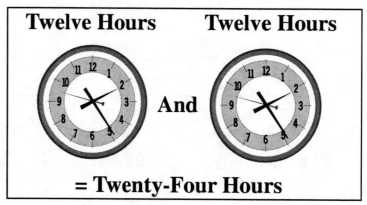

How To Teach All About Money

As with the concept of time, there are several steps to take when teaching a child about the concept of money. Since this is such a difficult concept to grasp well, it is important the therapist is sure that the child truly understands the idea of each activity before proceeding to the next step.

The therapist should introduce money by reading the money script with the child. The therapist and child should alternate reading lines. The script should be read every day until the child can anticipate the next line. The child will most probably not have grasped the concept of money; however, the concept will be more familiar to him/her.

In the same therapy sessions that use the money script, the money equation should also be used (immediately after the money script is read).

Once the child is very familiar with the money script and equation, then the therapist should introduce the child to the activities described in the Money Teaching Hierarchy IN THE SAME ORDER as indicated by the Money Teaching Hierarchy.

When the child grasps the material taught according to the Money Teaching Hierarchy, then it is time for the child to be introduced to the Concept of Enough Money. This set of activities is described in the Concept of Enough Money section which follows the Money Teaching Hierarchy.

The last stage of teaching about money is to have the child actually buy things and work with money. This should be relatively easy for the child if 1) s/he has mastered the Enough Money drills, and 2) the buying things with money activity has been acted out at home before going to the store.

Note: There are two money scripts, one that applies to the U.S.A. and one that applies to Canada. The child should only learn the script for the country in which s/he lives.

Why Teach All About Money?

The reason sequencing and comparing is so important is that without these skills, the child cannot fully grasp the concept of money. Without money concepts, it is difficult for the child to become an autonomous adult and protect him/herself from being taken advantage of economically. Money is a very difficult concept to completely grasp. It may take years for the child to completely understand the concept of money. These drills are designed to make explicit what is generally implicit, and thereby, make money concepts easier for the child to grasp.

About Money (U.S.A.)

When the child has mastered sequencing with numbers, s/he is ready to learn about money. This script is designed to be read with the child, emphasizing the words in bold as it is read. The script can also be read by the child and therapist alternating lines. The script should be in much larger format (on a full sheet of paper) to make it easier to read. Once the script is read, the therapist should explain the visual representation which follows (the money line). This must be done daily in order for the child to learn the script. Note: The therapist should use either the USA or the Canada money script, not both.

About Money (U.S.A.)

MONEY is something you **USE TO BUY THINGS.**

You **NEED MONEY** to **BUY FOOD** you see **IN SAFEWAY.**

You **NEED MONEY** to **BUY TOYS** you see **IN TOYS R US.**

You **NEED MONEY** to **BUY A HAMBURGER AND FRIES AT MCDONALDS.**

You **NEED MONEY** to **BUY CLOTHES** you see **AT TARGET.**

MONEY is something you **NEED TO DO SPECIAL THINGS.**

You **NEED MONEY** to **GO TO THE THEATER TO WATCH A MOVIE.**

You **NEED MONEY** to **GO TO THE ZOO.**

You **NEED MONEY** to **GO TO DISNEYLAND.**

You **NEED MONEY** to **FLY ON AN AIRPLANE.**

There are **DIFFERENT KINDS OF MONEY.**

COINS are **MONEY.**

A **PENNY, NICKEL, DIME, QUARTER, AND HALF-DOLLAR** are **COINS.**

They are all **KINDS OF MONEY.**

DOLLAR BILLS are **MONEY.**

A **ONE-DOLLAR, A FIVE-DOLLAR, A TEN-DOLLAR, AND A TWENTY-DOLLAR BILL are** all KINDS OF **MONEY.**

DIFFERENT KINDS OF MONEY have **DIFFERENT VALUES.**

DIFFERENT KINDS OF MONEY are **WORTH DIFFERENT AMOUNTS.**

Here is the **AMOUNT** each **KIND OF MONEY** is **WORTH.**

Here is the VALUE of each **KIND OF MONEY:**

A **PENNY** is **WORTH 1** or one cent. It is written in dollar notation as **$.01**

A **NICKEL** is **WORTH 5** or five cents. It is written in dollar notation as **$.05**

A **DIME** is **WORTH 10** or ten cents. It is written in dollar notation as **$.10**

A **QUARTER** is **WORTH 25** or twenty-five cents. It is written in dollar notation as $.25.

A **HALF-DOLLAR** is **WORTH 50** or fifty cents. It is written in dollar notation as **$.50**

A **ONE DOLLAR BILL** is **WORTH 100** or 100 cents. It is written in dollar notation as **$1.00**

A **FIVE DOLLAR BILL** is **WORTH five one-dollar bills.** It is written in dollar notation as **$5.00**

A **TEN DOLLAR BILL** is **WORTH ten one-dollar bills.** It is written in dollar notation as **$10.00**

A **TWENTY DOLLAR BILL** is **WORTH twenty one-dollar bills.** It is written in dollar notation as **$20.00**

About Money continued (USA)

This visual representation of the relative value of money should be introduced to the child after s/he has worked on the preceding script. These two tools complement each other and should always be presented together.

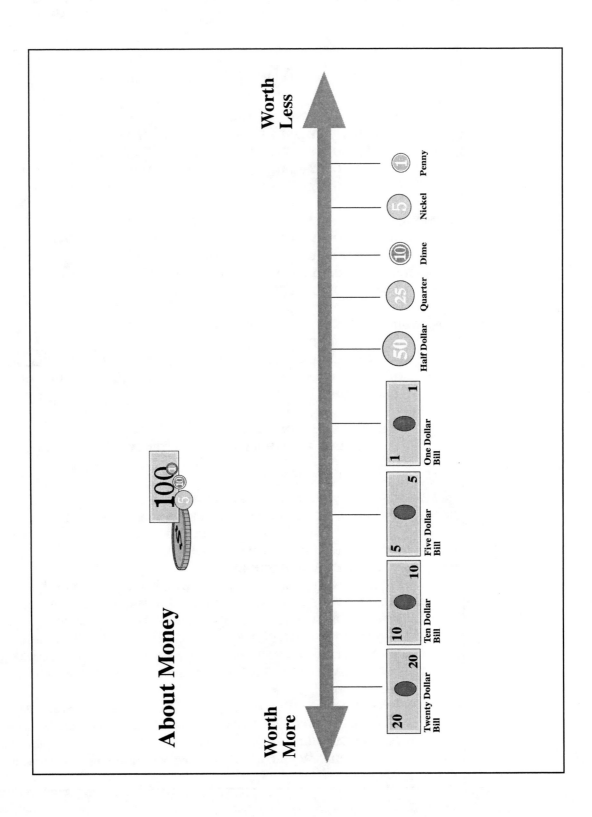

About Money (Canada)

When the child has mastered sequencing with numbers, s/he is ready to learn about money. This script is designed to be read with the child, emphasizing the words in bold as it is read. The script can also be read by the child and therapist alternating lines. The script should be in much larger format (on a full sheet of paper) to make it easier to read. Once the script is read, the therapist should explain the visual representation which follows. This must be done daily in order for the child to learn it. Note: Use either the USA or the Canada money script, not both.

About Money (Canada)

MONEY is something you **USE TO BUY THINGS.**

You **NEED MONEY** to **BUY FOOD** you see **IN SAFEWAY.**

You **NEED MONEY** to **BUY TOYS** you see **IN TOYS R US.**

You **NEED MONEY** to **BUY A HAMBURGER AND FRIES AT MCDONALDS.**

You **NEED MONEY** to **BUY CLOTHES** you see **AT THE BAY.**

MONEY is something you **NEED TO DO SPECIAL THINGS.**

You **NEED MONEY** to **GO TO THE THEATER TO WATCH A MOVIE.**

You **NEED MONEY** to **GO TO THE ZOO.**

You **NEED MONEY** to **GO TO DISNEYLAND.**

You **NEED MONEY** to **FLY ON AN AIRPLANE.**

There are **DIFFERENT KINDS OF MONEY.**

COINS ARE MONEY.

A **PENNY, NICKEL, DIME, QUARTER, HALF-DOLLAR, ONE DOLLAR, and TWO DOLLARS** are **COINS.**

They are all **KINDS OF MONEY.**

DOLLAR BILLS are **MONEY.**

A **FIVE-DOLLAR, A TEN-DOLLAR, AND A TWENTY-DOLLAR BILL** are all KINDS OF MONEY.

DIFFERENT KINDS OF MONEY have **DIFFERENT VALUES.**

DIFFERENT KINDS OF MONEY are **WORTH DIFFERENT AMOUNTS.**

Here is the **AMOUNT** each **KIND OF MONEY** is **WORTH.**

Here is the VALUE of each **KIND OF MONEY:**

A **PENNY** is **WORTH 1** or one cent. It is written in dollar notation as **$.01**

A **NICKEL** is **WORTH 5** or five cents. It is written in dollar notation as **$.05**

A **DIME** is **WORTH 10** or ten cents. It is written in dollar notation as **$.10**

A **QUARTER** is **WORTH 25** or twenty-five cents. It is written in dollar notation as **$.25**

A **HALF-DOLLAR** is **WORTH 50** or fifty cents. It is written in dollar notation as **$.50**

A **ONE DOLLAR COIN (LOONY)** is **WORTH 100 or 100 CENTS.** It is written in dollar notation as **$1.00**

A **TWO DOLLAR COIN** is **WORTH 200.** It is written in dollar notation as **$2.00**

A **FIVE DOLLAR BILL** is **WORTH five one-dollar coins.** It is written in dollar notation as **$5.00**

A **TEN DOLLAR BILL** is **WORTH ten one-dollar coins.** It is written in dollar notation as **$10.00**

A **TWENTY DOLLAR BILL** is **WORTH twenty one-dollar coins.** It is written in dollar notation as **$20.00**

About Money continued (Canada)

This visual representation of the relative value of money should be introduced to the child after s/he has worked on the preceding script. These two tools complement each other and should always be presented together.

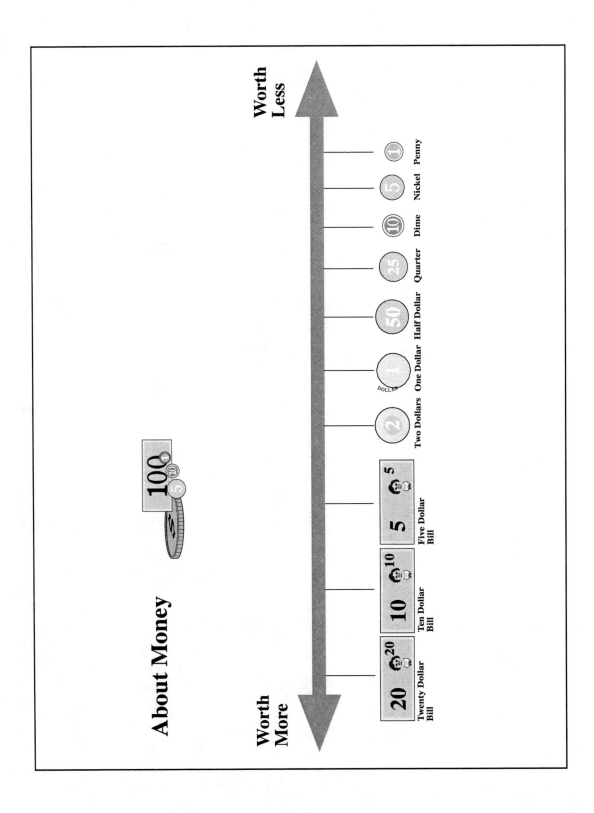

Money Equations

The money equations are another way to highlight the relative value of money and should be introduced to the child after s/he has worked on the money script and the visual representation that accompanies the money script and has learned the script well.

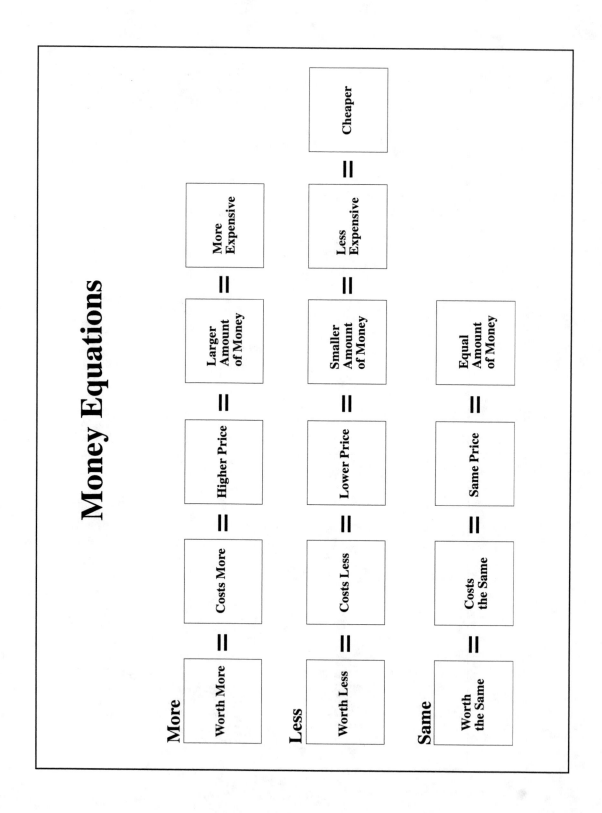

Money Equations

More

Worth More = Costs More = Higher Price = Larger Amount of Money = More Expensive

Less

Worth Less = Costs Less = Lower Price = Smaller Amount of Money = Less Expensive = Cheaper

Same

Worth the Same = Costs the Same = Same Price = Equal Amount of Money

Money Teaching Hierarchy

Prerequisite: The child must know the value of a coin based on how many cents it is worth (e.g. 1 penny = 1 cent, 1 nickel = 5 cents, 1 dime = 10 cents).

Note: Some children have a very difficult time learning about money using actual coins. If the child has particular difficulty with any of the drills described below, it is a good idea to introduce the concept using cards which have the names of the coins on them instead of using the coins themselves. Once the child learns how to do the drill using the cards, then the coins can be matched to the cards and the child can learn to count with the coins, making sure that the cards are in clear view. Eventually, the cards can be faded.

1. Sequencing Coins and Bills

a. Sequencing Coins

The first skill the child must learn is how to sequence coins in terms of their value. The therapist should show the child how to order the coins from the coin worth "less" and "least" to the coin worth "more" and "most" (i.e. penny, nickel, dime, quarter, and half-dollar). This skill should be taught using the cards provided in <u>Teach Me Language</u>.

First the therapist should put out a "more" card at one end of the table and a "less" card at the other. Then the therapist should sequence the coins for the child from the "more" card to the "less" card. Then the child should be asked to repeat the same sequence. It is important that the child learn to sequence horizontally (from one side of the table to the other) and vertically (from the top to the bottom), and from "less" and "least" to "more" and "most", and "more" and "most" to "less" and "least". Once the child can sequence the coins as described above, the therapist should replace "more" with "costs more" and "less" with "costs less".

Eventually, the therapist can teach the child that "costs more" means "higher price", and "costs less" means "lower price." The child needs to know that these are equivalent terms.

b. Sequencing Bills

The therapist should teach the child to sequence bills of different denominations from "least" to "most" (1$, 5$, $10, up to a $100 bill). First the therapist should sequence the cards for the child. The "most" card should be at one end of the sequence, and the "least" card at the other. Then the child should be asked to repeat the same sequence. This is generally easy for the child once s/he has learned to sequence coins.

c. Sequencing Coins and Bills

This skill is simply a combination of coin sequencing and bill sequencing taught prior to combining coins and bills. In this exercise, the child is asked to sequence the coins and bills from "least amount of money" to "most amount of money" up through $100.

d. Sequencing Work Sheet

Once the child can sequence using the cards and/or money, then it is time to introduce the "Sequencing and Ordering" work sheet in this section.

2. Comparing - Worth More/Worth Less

a. Comparing Coins

First, the therapist should have the child sequence the coins. Then the therapist should take two of the coins out of the sequence and ask the child which coin is worth either "more" or "less" (a quarter versus a nickel, a penny versus a dime, etc.). Once the child understands the relative worth of each coin by comparing the coins to each other, then the same should be done with bills.

b. Comparing Bills

Initially, the therapist should have the child sequence the bills. Then the therapist should take two of the bills out of the sequence and ask the child which bill is worth either "more" or "less" ($5 versus $10, $1 versus $20, etc.). Once the child understands the relative worth of each bill by comparing the bills to each other, then the same should be done with both coins and bills combined.

c. Comparing Coins and Bills

The therapist should set the exercise up by having the child sequence the coins and bills together. Then the therapist should take two of the money units out of the sequence and ask the child which is worth either "more" or "less" (a quarter versus a dollar, a dime versus 5 dollars, etc.). Once the child understands the relative worth of each money unit by comparing two money units to each other, then the same should be done with three money units (a quarter, a dollar, and 10 dollars).

d. Comparing Money Work Sheets

Once the child can compare both coins and bills using the cards and/or money, then it is time to introduce the "Comparing Money" work sheets in this section.

3. Counting - Different Amounts of Change

a. Counting Different Amounts of Coins

This exercise teaches the child to count change up to $1. The therapist must instruct the child to start with the coin that is worth the most first, and count accordingly, from the coins worth the most, to those worth the least. Starting with the coin that is worth the most is a very important concept the child must learn.

b. Counting Different Amounts of Bills

This exercise teaches the child to count bills using $1, $5, $10, $20, $100, up to $1000. The therapist should prompt the child to start with the bill that is worth the most, and count accordingly, from the bills worth the most to the least.

c. Counting Different Amounts of Bills and Coins

Once the child can count different amounts of coins and bills separately, it is time to have the child work on counting different amounts of money when both coins and bills are involved. The therapist should work incrementally on this skill at first, counting amounts from $1-$2, then $0-$2, then 0-$3 or $4. If the therapist introduces too large a span at once ($1 - $10) the child may have difficulty.

4. Equivalencies - Coins and Bills

Prerequisite: The child should be able to relate $1, $5, $10, and $20 bills to the value of a penny - i.e. $1 = 100 pennies. (There is no need to relate $50, $100 to pennies unless it is important for a specific child).

a. Equivalent Sets Using Coins

First, the therapist must teach the child that 1 nickel is the same as 5 pennies, 1 dime is the same as 10 pennies or 2 nickels, etc. The therapist should have the child match one coin by using other coins. For example, the child should learn that 5 pennies = 1 nickel by physically counting the pennies and placing them beside the nickel. For example, this can be taught by having the child match the nickel with 5 pennies. The child should be able to make equivalent sets from smaller coin values for a nickel, dime, quarter, half-dollar, and dollar bill (as in the example above). If the child has mastered the earlier sequencing skill (putting the coins in order, from "worth the least" to "worth the most"), s/he should be able to learn that each larger valued coin or dollar bill can be equally represented by using any number of combinations of coins of lesser value. The child does not need to know all the combinations, but should demonstrate understanding of the concept of equivalent sets of money/coins.

Note: Some children have difficulties using actual coins or pictures of coins. If the child is having difficulty with the concept, cards that have the names of the coins on them can be used instead. Then the child learns that the dime card equals 10 penny cards, and the quarter card equals two dime cards and one nickel card. Eventually, the cards can be replaced with coins once the concept of equivalent worth is understood.

b. Equivalent Sets with Bills

Prerequisite: In order to understand equivalencies with bills, the child must know how to count by 5's, 10's, 20's, 25's, 50's, and 100's.

First, the therapist must teach the child different ways to make a variety of amounts using bills. For example, a 5 dollar bill is the same as 5 one dollar bills (or 1 dollar coins); 1 ten dollar bill is the same as 2 five dollar bills or 10 one dollar bills. The therapist should have the child match one bill by using other bills. The child should be able to make equivalent sets (as in the example above) from smaller bills to larger bills. If the child has mastered the earlier sequencing skill (putting the bills in order from "worth the least" to "worth the most"), s/he should be able to learn that each larger valued bill can be equally represented by using any number of combinations of bills of lesser value.

c. Equivalent Sets with Coins and Bills

When given an amount of money, the child should be able to select different combinations of dollars and coins to make an equivalent set. This is a good time to introduce the concept of "same amount". The child will need this skill to be able to determine which amount of money is "more", "less" or "the same" when judging between two sets. If the child has been able to make equivalent sets with coins and bills separately, s/he should be able to combine these two skills, as long as the therapist proceeds in stages.

5. Comparing - Sets of Money

a. Sets of Coins up to $1

The therapist prepares this exercise by creating small sets of coins, each set of coins amounting to less than $1. Then the therapist has the child choose between two groups of coins, indicating which group is "worth more" (or "worth the most"), and which group is "worth less" (or "worth the least"). For example, one set of coins is made up of 1 nickel, and 2 dimes. The second set of coins contains 1 quarter and 1 nickel. The child must choose the second set of coins over the first. The child may incorrectly choose the set of coins with the most coins, rather than the set that is worth more. If this occurs, the therapist should make sure the child adds up each set before comparing the two.

b. Sets of Bills up to $1000

The therapist prepares this exercise in much the same way as she prepares the coins. She must create small sets of bills, each set of bills can reach a maximum of $1000. Then the therapist has the child choose between two groups of bills, indicating which group is "worth more" (or "worth the most"), and which group is "worth less" (or "worth the least").

c. Sets of Bills and Coins

This step is a combination of the prior two steps. The child must determine which set of bills and coins, up to $1000, is more and which is less. The therapist should work incrementally with this concept, and eventually have the child learn to compare 3 sets of money. When working with large bills, their are to many combinations to have the child count them all; therefore, the therapist can use a variety of combinations until the child understands the concept.

d. Money Questions (Auditory)

Once the child understands equivalencies using the cards and/or money, then it is time to introduce the "Money Questions" work sheet in this section.

6. Making Change

a. Making Change with Coins for 1 Item Purchased

In this exercise, the child learns to give back change for an item which costs up to $1. The therapist should have the child be the "cashier". The child is given an item and some change. S/he must first state the cost of the item. Then s/he should count back change starting with the price of the item. Then the child should count, giving the proper coins, up to the amount s/he is given. For example, let us say that the item costs 35 cents. The child is given 50 cents. The child should say, "It costs 35 cents." Then s/he should count, "45, 50", and give the person a dime and a nickel. The therapist should stress the use of the most "efficient" coins for making change (i.e. using a dime and a nickel rather than 15 pennies).

b. Making Change with Coins for 2+ Items Purchased

This exercise is done in exactly the same way as the exercise above; however, in this case the child is given two items which together cost less than $1. In this case, the child needs to learn that s/he must first add the cost of each item, and use that total as the place to begin counting back change. In other words, the child needs to understand the concept of "total cost". If this is difficult, have the child add two purchases together on paper and then use the written total to make change.

c. Making Change with Coins and Bills for Large Purchases

This exercise teaches the child to make change with coins and bills together. Initially, the therapist should make the item cost exactly 5 dollars, for example. Once the child can give back change using bills only, then bills and coins can be combined. If the child has learned steps a. and b., this task should become easier. It is important the therapist works incrementally with the amounts to make sure the child understands how to make change using coins and bills at the same time. Eventually the child should be able to make change when given a number of items which add up to $1000. The therapist should "spot check" this skill using various amounts and a number of items to make sure the child has grasped the concept.

The exercises which involve making change can be approached through role-playing with a peer. "Kiddy" menus from restaurants or the "Let's Go Shopping" game are both highly motivating ways to practice this skill.

7. Reading and Writing Prices

In addition to the above tasks, the child needs to be able to read prices and write prices when given the verbal amount (e.g. "write 4 dollars, fifty-nine cents in dollar notation"). An more difficult task the child must eventually learn is to translate coins into dollar notation (e.g. 74 cents = $0.74) and translate coin names into dollar notation (e.g., 7 dimes and 4 pennies in dollar notation = $0.74). This should not be introduced until the child's typically developing peers are taught the skill.

Cards For Teaching Money

These are reproducible money cards to be used as explained in the Money Hierarchy on the previous pages. These cards can be photocopied onto card stock to ensure their durability. Several cards of each denomination should be made in order to have enough cards to make change.

penny	**nickel**
dime	**quarter**
half dollar	**1 dollar**
2 dollars	**5 dollars**

For Canadian children only

Cards For Teaching Money

These are reproducible money cards to be used as explained in the Money Hierarchy on the previous pages. These cards can be photocopied onto card stock to ensure their durability. Several cards of each denomination should be made in order to have enough cards to make change.

10 dollars	**500 dollars**
20 dollars	**1000 dollars**
50 dollars	**costs more**
100 dollars	**costs less**

Cards For Teaching Money

These are reproducible money cards to be used as explained in the Money Hierarchy on the previous pages. These cards can be photocopied onto card stock to ensure their durability. Several cards of each denomination should be made in order to have enough cards to make change.

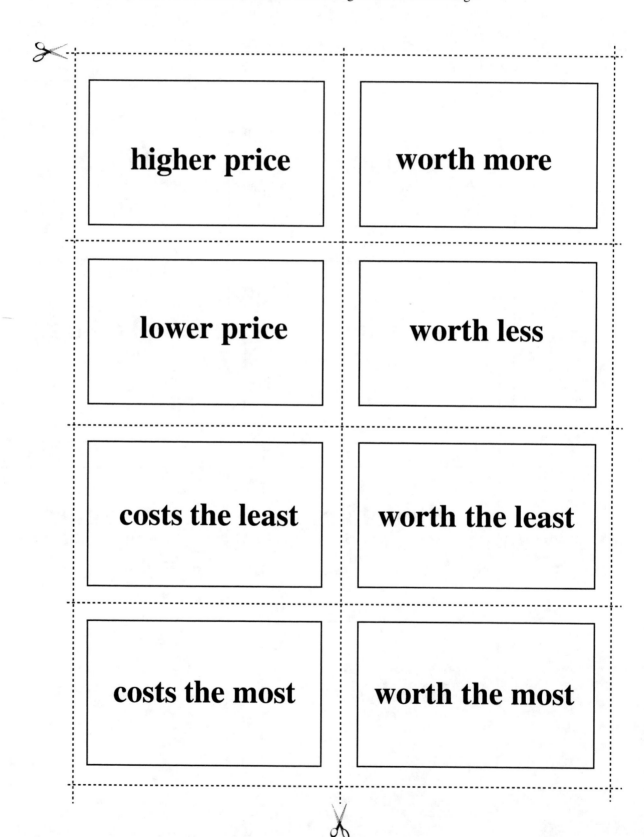

higher price

worth more

lower price

worth less

costs the least

worth the least

costs the most

worth the most

Comparing Money - Sheet 1

The money comparison exercise gives the child practice at looking at relative amounts and discerning their relative value. It is important that the child have this concept firmly internalized before s/he can use money independently.

Comparing Money - Sheet 1

Look at each amount of money.
Circle the amount that:

is more $1.89   ($2.00) $1.99

is least $.57   ($.36) $1.20

is the higher price $.53 $.77   ($1.00)

is the lower price $2.00   ($.02) $1.02

Comparing Money - Sheet 2

This second money comparison exercise is much harder than the first because the amounts are larger and more complex. It is important for the child to be able to do this drill very easily before the concepts of "enough money" and "change back" are introduced.

Comparing Money - Sheet 2

Look at each amount of money.
Circle the amount that:

is more	$1.88 $2.12 ($3.15)	$ .77 ($1.73) $ .99	$ .64 $ .06 ($1.01)
is less	$12.80 $16.40 ($10.90)	($2.00) $2.50 $2.11	($3.06) $3.10 $3.20
is more	$22.00 $8.96 ($34.11)	$3.11 ($8.15) $6.27	$2.99 ($3.99) $ .99

Sequencing And Ordering

This exercise has the child order numbers or money in a particular sequence. In this example, the therapist concentrates on the concept of relative prices.

Sequencing and Ordering

Read each direction and order the _numbers and prices_ by writing 1, 2, 3, and 4 in the correct boxes.

bigger number to smaller number	6	98	76	10
	3	1	2	4

higher price to lower price	$2.50	$99.76	$200.00	$350.00
	4	3	2	1

larger number to smaller number	22	360	1,672	912
	4	3	1	2

more $ to less $ lower price	$50.00	$80.00	$60.00	$20.00
	3	1	2	4

Concept Of Enough Money

Prerequisite: The child must understand the concept of more and less with amounts of money under $1 before the "Enough Money" concept is taught.

In order to teach the concept of "Enough Money" the therapist needs to make or buy cards that have pictures of coins on them, each card with a variety of coins. The amount of each card is different. The card with the highest amount is 75 cents. The therapist can create cards of this type by taping groups of coins to individual cards or buying Money Match Me cards (available at any teacher supply store). To set up this activity, the therapist must place "amount" cards on the table in the following order:

less than enough	the same amount	more than enough

1. Enough Money Using Coin Cards

The therapist should put out one of the coin cards and proceed as follows:
   a) first, the child should count the change on the card and tell the therapist how much money there is.
   b) second, the therapist should alternate, giving the child either the correct number of coins, OR the correct change to match the card, but **withholding** 1 to 2 coins.
   c) third, the therapist has the child match his/her coins to the card (putting the actual coins on top of the coins depicted on the card). She then asks the child, "Do you have enough money?" Once the child understands the matching task, the therapist can say, "An ice-cream costs 75 cents. Do you have enough money to buy the ice-cream?"

The child should tell the therapist if he does or does not have enough money. If all the coins are matched, then the child can answer "yes" and put the matched set below the card that says "the same amount". If s/he is one or two coins short, then the child should put the matched set below the "less than enough" card. The child should be asked, "How much do you need?" The answer to this question is simple at this stage because the "missing" amount is represented on the card; it is the total of whichever coins are unmatched.

Note: The therapist must make sure the child uses a complete sentence to answer (this may initially have to be prompted). If s/he has enough money, the child should give one of the following answers: "Yes, I have enough money; I have the same amount", "Yes, I have enough; I have more than enough money," or "No, I don't have enough money. I have less than enough money."

2. Enough Money Using Written Amounts of Money

Step 1 should be repeated using cards that do not show pictures of coins on them but, rather, have written amounts of money under $1 on each card. The child should be given the correct or incorrect (too little) change as in Step 1. The therapist should instruct the child to count the amount of money given to him/her. Then the therapist should ask the child, "Do you have enough money?". If the child answers, "No", the therapist then asks him/her how much more s/he needs.

Note: The child may not easily transfer money skills to this task since there is nothing for the child to match. The child will have to know that his/her amount is "more", "the same" or "less" than the written price. If necessary, the therapist can place the correct amount of coins next to the written amount (as a matched set), then give the child the money and have him/her answer the question, "Do you have enough money?" The child can look at his/her set and compare it with the written amount and the coins next to it. The child should be able to answer the therapist's question without directly matching the coins on top as in Step 1.

If the child does not have enough money, then s/he must decide how much extra money s/he needs. This is difficult when the written amount is the only information the child has. The child must be taught to:

a. count up from the amount s/he has to the amount s/he needs. The therapist should give the child coins to do this. The child's set of coins should be next to the written amount on the card. The child should tell the therapist how much s/he has and how much s/he needs (for example, "I have 45 cents, but I need 52 cents").

b. Once the child states the amount s/he needs, the child can take the correct coins and count up to the amount on the card. The child should slide these new coins under the card so that s/he does not confuse the new coins with the original set. The amount of the coins s/he slid under the card is how much more s/he needs. It is better to have the child figure out the amount s/he needs this way rather than just subtracting in her/his head (which is ultimately what s/he must learn to do). Using this visual technique, the steps the child must go through will become clearer. In addition, when the child begins to work on counting back change, s/he will have a good foundation on how to do so.

3. Written Amounts up to $100 or More

If the child can grasp the concept of "enough" money up to $100, s/he probably has grasped the concept. With larger amounts, the child will need to subtract using a pen and paper. The therapist must make sure that the child understands the concept of "how much **more** do you need?", before assuming the child has grasped the concept of "Enough Money."

4. Work Sheets

Once the child can do Steps 1 through 3, then the first "Do I Have Enough Money" work sheet can be introduced. This work sheet targets the concepts of "having the correct amount of money" or "needing more money". Once the child can do this work sheet, the second "Do I Have Enough Money" work sheet can be introduced. The second work sheet focuses on the additional skill of determining how much change the child should receive. Once the child can do the second work sheet, then the "Buying Things and Working With Money" work sheet can be introduced. This is the most complex of all the "Money" work sheets. If the child masters this work sheet, s/he has the foundation required to use money independently.

Do I Have Enough Money? - Sheet 1

This exercise is designed to give the child the tools s/he needs to grasp the concept of "enough money". The therapist should go through the drill several times with the child until s/he understands the concept. The next step is to play "store" with the therapist and then with a peer. Once the child can do the sheet relatively well and can pretend play "store", the s/he can be taken to a restaurant or store. The child should order something and compute the change s/he should receive. By making this realistic, the child will understand and be motivated to use this skill, especially to make sure s/he has enough money for the purchase of choice.

Do I Have Enough Money ? - Sheet 1

When you want to buy something, you have to figure out if you have enough money to buy it.

Item	Cost	Money I have
Pancakes at Denny's (item)	$1.79	1 dollar 1 quarter 2 dimes

Total Money I have ⟶ $ 1.45

Do I have enough money to buy ___pancakes___ ?   **Yes / No**
                                      (item)   (circle one)

Which do I have? (circle one)

- Less Than Enough

- More Than Enough

- Just Enough
  (the same amount as the cost)

If I have **less than enough money,** how much **more money** do I need?

Cost of ___pancakes___ (item)	$ 1.79
How money do I have	$ 1.45
How Much More Money I Need	$ .34

Do I Have Enough Money - Sheet 2

This more difficult exercise is designed to teach the child 1) whether or not s/he has enough money, and 2) when s/he has too much money, how much change s/he should get back. The therapist should go through the drill several times with the child until s/he understands the concept of "getting change back". Once the child can do this drill easily, then s/he should start incorporating this skill into his/her daily life (every time the child goes to a store or restaurant).

Do I Have Enough Money ? - Sheet 2

When you want to buy something, you have to figure out if you have enough money to buy it.

Item	**Cost**	**Money I have**
Pancakes at Denny's	$1.79	1 dollar
(item)		2 quarters
		4 dimes

Total Money I have ⟶ $ 1.90

Do I have enough money to buy __pancakes__ ? **Yes** / **No**
                                    (item)   (circle one)

Which do I have? (circle one)

- Less Than Enough

- More Than Enough

- Just Enough
  (the same amount
  as the cost)

If I have **less than enough money,** how much **more money** do I need?		If I have **more than enough money,** how much **change** do I get back?	
Cost of _____ (item)	$	How money do I have	$ 1.90
How money do I have	$	Cost of __pancakes__ (item)	$ 1.79
How Much More Money I Need	$	How Much Change Do I Get Back?	$ .11

Buying Things & Working With Money

This exercises builds on the previous exercises. In this exercise the child learns to use money when there is more than one item being bought. Incorporated into this exercise is the concept of "enough money", "change back", and "total cost".

Buying Things and Working With Money

You want to buy these things: Cost:

1. _donuts_ $ _.35_
     _____(item)_____
2. _cupcakes_ (item) $ _.50_
     _____(item)_____
3. _____ $ _____
     _____(item)_____

What is the **TOTAL COST?** ⟶ | $ _.85_ |

What is the largest bill you will need?   (circle one)

(**$1**) $5 $10 $20

If you have $ _.50_ , will you have enough money to buy the items?   _No_

If you have $ _1.00_ , will you have enough money to buy the items?   _Yes_

If you have $ _1.00_ , will you have more or less money than you need? _More_

If you have $ _.50_ , will you have more or less money than you need? _Less_

If you want to give the cashier the **EXACT AMOUNT OF MONEY,** what would you give her?

Number of bills or coins: _____ dollars = $ _____
                          __3__ quarters = $ _.75_
                          __1__ dimes   = $ _.10_
                          _____ nickels = $ _____
                          _____ pennies = $ _____

TOTAL ⟶ | $ _.85_ |

If you gave the cashier $ _1.00_ , how much change would you get back?

Amount you give the cashier $ _1.00_

The cost of the items (subtract)   − $ _.85_

Change you should get back ⟶ | $ _.15_ |

Money Questions (Auditory)

This exercise has the child listen and then answer questions which ask about the relative worth of money. These questions should be customized to the individual child so that the questions relate to his/her life. This auditory drill should not be done with the child until the preceding written exercises on relative value of money are understood completely by the child.

Auditory Money Questions

Which is worth the most, _$1.00 or $2.00_ ?

Which is worth the least, _$.50 or $.75_ ?

Which is the higher price, _$.2.50 or $3.25_ ?

Which is the lower price, _$1.25 or $1.99_ ?

Which costs more, _a pencil or five pencil_ ?

Which costs more, your school lunch or a candy bar?

Which costs less, a coke or a happy meal?

How To Teach Sequencing Parts of the Day

The child should learn the basic idea of sequencing from his/her own schedule. The therapist should introduce this exercise by choosing a very easy sequence i.e. answering the phone. The therapist should teach the child by using the words, "First", "Next", and "Last". i.e. "First, the phone rings. Next we pick up the phone. Last, we say, "Hello, this is John". This should be acted out until the child understands the idea of this sequence. Once the child has an introductory understanding of sequencing activities, the next step is to teach sequencing with the "Task, Plan, and Sequence" cards. The therapist puts the three cards out on the table. Under the TASK card, she needs to put the title of the activity such as "Getting Ready for School". Under the "PLAN" card, she puts the cards with the medium size typeface i.e. what, when, where, how, money, decide, how many. Under the "SEQUENCE" card, the child must put the action cards into the correct sequence. Then, if the child is verbal, s/he must read the task card out loud. Using the cards in the correct order as a prompt, the child must say, for example, "First, I get dressed. Next, I eat breakfast. Last I get my school bag (or backpack)". The child may need considerable prompting at first; however, once s/he memorizes the sequence, s/he should be able to do this task quite easily. The therapist should introduce all the cards slowly, being careful to set the child up for success.

Once the child can easily sequence parts of his/her day using the cards, the next step is to have the child sequence these same activities with word cards only. Over the years, the sequences should become more complex, and the therapist can add more steps as needed.

Why Sequence Part Of The Day?

The goal of this exercise is not for the child to memorize particular sequences; rather, this exercise makes sequencing explicit. The drill is designed to work on internalizing the concept of sequencing. The TASK, PLAN, SEQUENCE structure makes it easier for the child to notice sequences in his/her natural environment and thereby, organize them into the correct order.

Sequences The Child Should Learn

The sequences listed below are common sequences that most every child should learn. Most sequences, however, should be customized to the child's own schedule and weekly activities.

Getting Ready for School

get out of bed
get dressed
eat breakfast
brush your teeth
go to school

Brushing Teeth

put water on the toothbrush
put toothpaste on the toothbrush
brush your teeth
rinse your mouth with water

Eating Out in a Restaurant

go to the restaurant
waited to be seated
order food from the waiter
eat the food
pay for the food

Answering the Phone

the phone rings
pick up the phone
say, "Hello, this is John."

Going to buy Groceries

make a list of what you need
go to the store
put food in your grocery cart
pay the clerk for the food

Crossing the Street

stop at the curb or street corner
look right and left for cars
listen for cars
walk across the street when it's safe

Sequencing Parts Of The Day

This is an example of the sequencing exercise using the Task, Plan, Sequence cards. The child is taught to organize the cards as below. This drill visually structures the critical thinking process of thinking about an activity, asking oneself questions to plan for the activity, and then explicitly sequencing the activity.

Task	Plan	Sequence

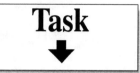

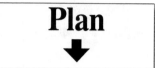

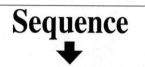

Going to the Store

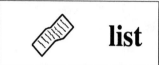 go to the store

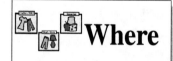 list

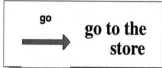 get what you need

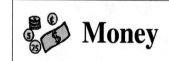 Money

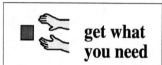 pay the cashier or clerk

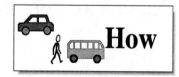 How

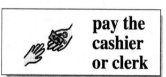

Sequencing Parts Of The Day

These cards are designed to be used to teach the child how to sequence parts of his/her day. Explanations on how to use these cards precede this page.

Master
Task
Card

Task ⬇

Master
Plan
Card

Plan ⬇

Master
Sequence
Card

Sequence ⬇

The Picture Communication Symbols on the following pages are used with permission © Mayer-Johnson Co., 1981-1995. To order a complete set of Mayer-Johnson picture communication symbols, telephone (619) 550-0084.

Sequencing Parts Of The Day

These cards are designed to teach the child how to sequence parts of his/her day. Explanations on how to use these cards precede this page. These particular cards are Task - Plan - Sequence Cards for Getting Ready for School

A Task
Card

Getting Ready for School

A Plan
Card

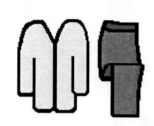 **what**

A Plan
Card

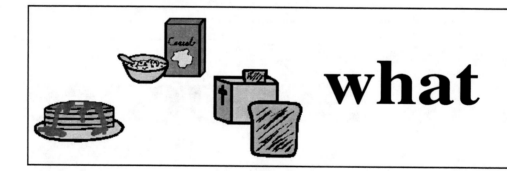

A Plan
Card

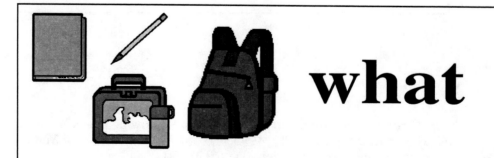

Picture Communication Symbols are used with permission© Mayer-Johnson Co., 1981-1995. Ph.:(619)550-0084

Sequencing Parts Of The Day

These cards are designed to teach the child how to sequence parts of his/her day. Explanations on how to use these cards precede this page. These particular cards are Task - Plan - Sequence Cards for Getting Ready for School.

A Plan
Card

 **when**

A Sequence
Card

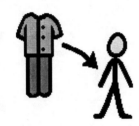 **get dressed**

A Sequence
Card

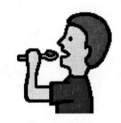 **eat breakfast**

A Sequence
Card

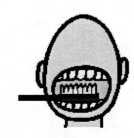 **brush your teeth**

Sequencing Parts Of The Day

These cards are designed to teach the child how to sequence parts of his/her day. Explanations on how to use these cards precede this page. These particular cards are Task - Plan - Sequence Cards for Getting Ready for School

A Sequence
Card

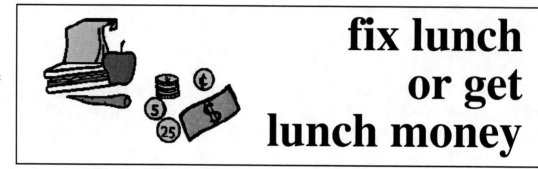

fix lunch or get lunch money

A Sequence
Card

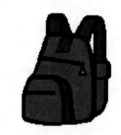

get your backpack

A Sequence
Card

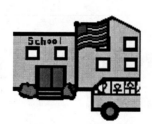

go to school

Sequencing Parts Of The Day

These cards are designed to help teach the child how to sequence parts of his/her day. Explanations on how to use these cards precede this page. These particular cards are Task - Plan - Sequence Cards for Ordering Food at a Fast Food Restaurant

A Task
Card

Ordering Food at a Fast Food Restaurant

A Plan
Card

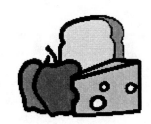 **what**

A Plan
Card

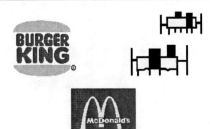 **where**

A Plan
Card

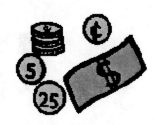 **money**

Picture Communication Symbols are used with permission© Mayer-Johnson Co., 1981-1995. Ph.:(619)550-0084

Sequencing Parts Of The Day

These cards are designed to be used to teach the child how to sequence parts of his/her day. Explanations on how to use these cards precede this page. These particular cards are Task - Plan - Sequence Cards for Ordering Food at a Fast Food Restaurant.

A Plan
Card

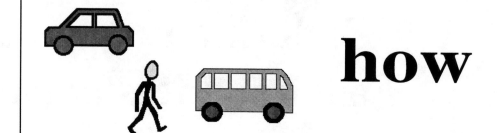

how

A Sequence
Card

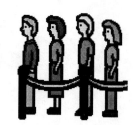

**stand in line
to order**

A Sequence
Card

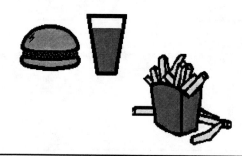

**order your
food**

A Sequence
Card

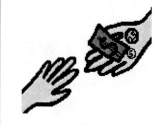

**pay for
your food**

Sequencing Parts Of The Day

These cards are designed to teach the child how to sequence parts of his/her day. Explanations on how to use these cards precede this page. These particular cards are Task - Plan - Sequence Cards for Ordering Food at a Fast Food Restaurant

A Sequence Card

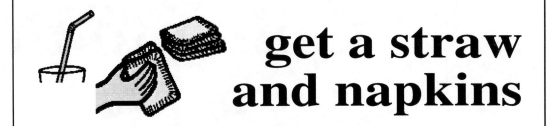 **get a straw and napkins**

A Sequence Card

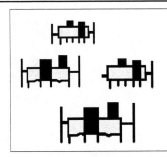 **find a table and sit down**

A Sequence Card

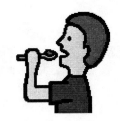 **eat your food**

A Sequence Card

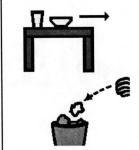 **clear your table & throw away your garbage**

Picture Communication Symbols are used with permission© Mayer-Johnson Co., 1981-1995. Ph.:(619)550-0084

Sequencing Parts Of The Day

These cards are designed to teach the child how to sequence parts of his/her day. Explanations on how to use these cards precede this page. These particular cards are Task - Plan - Sequence Cards for Going to the Store.

A Task
Card

Going to the Store

A Plan
Card

 **list**

A Plan
Card

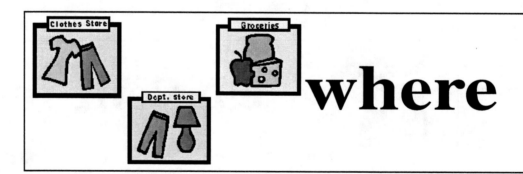 **where**

A Plan
Card

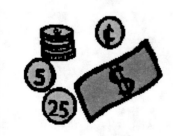 **money**

Sequencing Parts Of The Day

These cards are designed to teach the child how to sequence parts of his/her day. Explanations on how to use these cards precede this page. These particular cards are Task - Plan - Sequence Cards for Going To the Store.

A Plan
Card

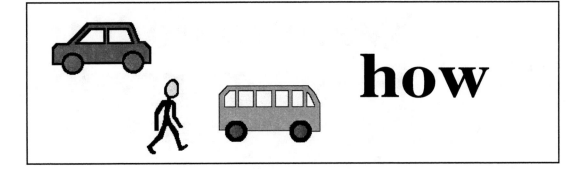

how

A Sequence
Card

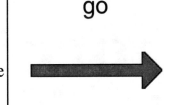

go to the store

A Sequence
Card

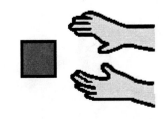

get what you need

A Sequence
Card

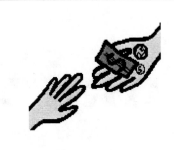

pay the cashier or clerk

Sequencing Parts Of The Day

These cards are designed to teach the child how to sequence parts of his/her day. Explanations on how to use these cards precede this page. These particular cards are Task - Plan - Sequence Cards for: What to do if there is an emergency at home.

A Task
Card

What to do if there is an emergency at home

A Plan
Card

emergency!

911

decide

A Plan
Card

help

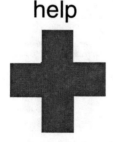

decide

A Plan
Card

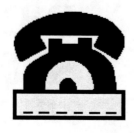

dial 911

Sequencing Parts Of The Day

These cards are designed to teach the child how to sequence parts of his/her day. Explanations on how to use these cards precede this page. These particular cards are Task - Plan - Sequence Cards for What To Do if There is an Emergency at Home.

A Sequence
Card

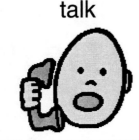

talk

Tell your name. Say, "hello, this is _____."

A Sequence
Card

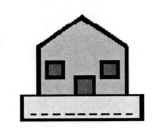

Tell your address. Say, "I live at _____."

A Sequence
Card

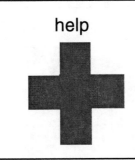

help

Say, "I need help."

A Sequence
Card

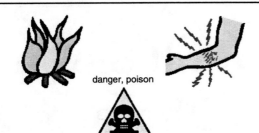

danger, poison

Tell what happened

Picture Communication Symbols are used with permission© Mayer-Johnson Co., 1981-1995. Ph.:(619)550-0084

Sequencing Parts Of The Day

These cards are designed to teach the child how to sequence parts of his/her day. Explanations on how to use these cards precede this page. These particular cards are Task - Plan - Sequence Cards for: Taking a Bath.

A Task Card

Taking a Bath

A Plan Card

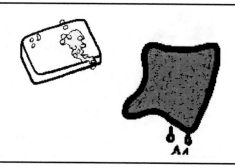

what
(for during the bath)

A Plan Card

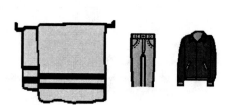

what
(for after the bath)

A Sequence Card

fill the bathtub with warm water

Sequencing Parts Of The Day

These cards are designed to teach the child how to sequence parts of his/her day. Explanations on how to use these cards precede this page. These particular cards are Task - Plan - Sequence Cards for: Taking a Bath.

A Sequence Card

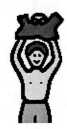

take off your clothes

A Sequence Card

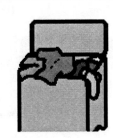

put your dirty clothes in the clothes hamper

A Sequence Card

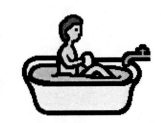

get in the bathtub

A Sequence Card

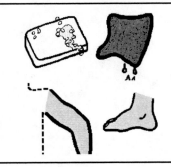

wash yourself with a washcloth and soap

Sequencing Parts Of The Day

These cards are designed to teach the child how to sequence parts of his/her day. Explanations on how to use these cards precede this page. These particular cards are Task - Plan - Sequence Cards for: Taking a Bath.

A Sequence
Card

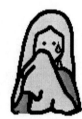 **get out of the tub and dry off with a towel**

A Sequence
Card

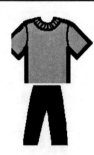 **put on your pajamas**

Sequencing Parts Of The Day

These cards are designed to teach the child how to sequence parts of his/her day. Explanations on how to use these cards precede this page. These particular cards are Task - Plan - Sequence Cards for: Setting the Table.

A Task
Card

Setting the Table

A Plan
Card

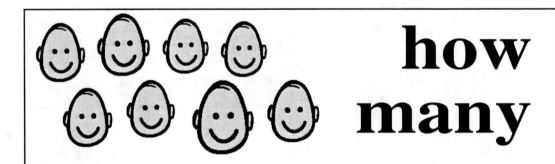

how
many

A Plan
Card

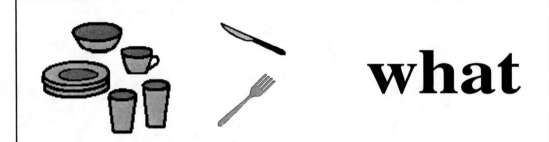

what

A Sequence
Card

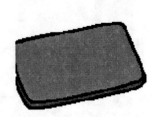

put place mats
on the table

Sequencing Parts Of The Day

These cards are designed to teach the child how to sequence parts of his/her day. Explanations on how to use these cards precede this page. These particular cards are Task - Plan - Sequence Cards for: Setting the Table.

A Sequence
Card

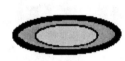

put plates on the place mats

A Sequence
Card

put napkins on the left side of the plates

A Sequence
Card

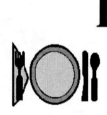

put a fork, knife, and spoon next to each plate

A Sequence
Card

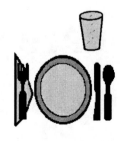

put a cup above each place setting

Picture Communication Symbols are used with permission© Mayer-Johnson Co., 1981-1995. Ph.:(619)550-0084

How To Teach Note-Taking

Using the simple sentences supplied on the following page, the therapist is to slowly read the sentence aloud. The child is instructed to write down the key words. The therapist then has the child retell the full sentence (or full idea) based on the notes s/he took. If the child has difficulty grasping the idea of note-taking, the therapist should show the child by demonstrating the notes she takes from the sentence she reads aloud. At first, the therapist should emphasize the words that she thinks are important to write down in order to be able to retrieve the full sentence. For example, the therapist should read, "the LION has a MANE", and the child should write down: Lion   Mane. Then the child should be able to say "the Lion has a Mane" based on the notes s/he takes. If the child can retrieve the information taking notes in a way that the therapist would not (writing down different key words) the child should not be corrected if the child's way of taking notes appears to work for him/her. However, if the child cannot retrieve the sentence or general idea, then the therapist should suggest additional or different words to be written down.

The first step in teaching note taking is to train the child to recognize key words in a sentence. Once the child understands the type of words that s/he is to write down, then the type of paragraphs used to teach note taking can be expanded. To introduce this exercise, the therapist should read three simple, unrelated sentences. The first type of sentence is included in the following pages in the Introductory section. Once the child masters these sentences, the therapist should go to the easiest story comprehension books (The Reading Milestones Series is an example of this) and have the child take notes on three related sentences in a story. In addition, the therapist could have the child take notes from factual material such as the animal paragraphs. As the child becomes good at note-taking, the material should GRADUALLY become more challenging. The eventual goal is to have the child be able to take simple notes from what the teacher is saying so that the child can look back at notes to understand what the teacher requires from him/her.

Note: The difficult note-taking is included to show how hard this drill can become. The examples of difficult material we provide will take years for the child to master. This material is difficult because the sentences include high level vocabulary and the excerpts are from fairy tales, which children with developmental delays generally find difficult to comprehend.

Why Teach Note-Taking?

The ability to take notes is important even though it may seem that in second or third grade this would be an inappropriate skill to teach. The idea is to have the child take notes and then use those notes to understand orally given directions. For example, if the teacher gives three instructions in fast succession, the child only needs to write down the key words without understanding what the teacher said. Then the child can read from the notes and know what is required. Another purpose of note-taking is to focus the child's attention on what the teacher is saying instead of becoming lost among all the different sounds in the classroom. Even if the child is unable to retrieve all the information given to him verbally, at least s/he has something to rely upon and is focused on the task at hand.

Key Word Sentences For Note-Taking (1)

This exercise is designed to improve the child's listening skills. The therapist should read one group of sentences per therapy session and teach the child to take notes only using the key words in the sentence. At first the therapist should pause after each sentence. Eventually the therapist should read the sentences at a normal pace without large pauses after each sentence. Then the child should be able to recall what was said. These beginning sentences have been chosen with the assumption that the child has already learned all about animals and occupation. The idea is to begin with factual information the child knows about. When reading the sentences to the child, they should be read slowly and with emphasis on the key words. Once the child understands the concept of note-taking, the emphasis should be toned down to replicate the intonation of a teacher.

Note: The sentences presented are examples of the kinds of sentences the child should work on at the various levels. The therapist will have to augment sentences since this exercise should be done daily over the course of years with different sentences each time.

Key Word Sentences For Note Taking (Introduction)

☐ 1. A horse is a mammal.
2. A duck is a kind of bird.
3. A ladybug is a kind of insect.
4. A frog is an amphibian.
5. A snake is a reptile.

☐ 1. Doctors take care of sick people.
2. Dentists take care of your teeth.
3. Carpenters build houses.
4. Chefs cook food.
5. Fire fighters put out fires.

☐ 1. A lion eats meat.
2. A giraffe eats twigs & leaves.
3. A bird eats worms.
4. A penguin eats fish.
5. A monkey eats fruit, insects and plants.

☐ 1. Farmers grow food.
2. A fireman works at a fire station.
3. Chefs work in a hotel or restaurant.
4. A carpenter works outside.
5. A dentist works in an office.

☐ 1. Lions live in Africa.
2. Tigers live in Asia.
3. Elephants live where it is hot.
4. Birds live in nests in the trees.
5. Monkeys live in the jungle.

☐ 1. Doctors use many special tools.
2. Carpenters use a saw, and a hammer.
3. Chefs use pots and pans, and a stove or oven.
4. Fire fighters use on axe, a hose and water.
5. Farmers use tractors and other machines.

☐ 1. Bears sleep all winter.
2. Kangaroos have gray or red fur.
3. Insects have six legs.
4. Mammals have a backbone.
5. Ladybugs have two pairs of wings.

☐ 1. Farmers gather eggs from the chickens.
2. Fire fighters wear special clothes.
3. Chefs wear a white hat or an apron.
4. Carpenters wear old clothes when they work.
5. A dentist will tell you to brush your teeth.

Key Word Sentences For Note Taking (2)

Once the child can take notes relatively well (based on the preceding note taking sheet), then it is time to introduce note taking using paragraphs that are not factual in nature, but rather, have a story to tell. This is much more difficult for the child since there is no prior knowledge that the child can rely upon. The therapist should start off slowly reading one group of sentences a session. If this is too difficult for the child, the therapist can begin by reading one sentence at a time until the child can master three sentences. The most difficult sentences are longer and have some words that the child will not know. The idea is for the child to get a general idea of what is happening but not to be able to repeat this sentence back verbatim. Once the child becomes proficient at note-taking (which may take years), it will help him/her in the classroom when the teacher gives group instruction (which occurs in all grades).

Note: The sentences presented are examples of the kinds of sentences the child should work on at the various levels. The therapist will have to augment sentences since this exercise should be done daily over the course of years using different sentences each time.

Key Word Sentences For Note Taking (2) Easy

☐ Sue bought some candy.
Then she walked home.
Sue gave the candy to Jim.

☐ The girls went to the circus.
They laughed at the clown.
The clown was riding a bike.

☐ The children sat on the hill.
They opened the picnic basket.
In the basket was cake.

☐ Dan loves to see movies.
He goes to the movies every Saturday.
Dan likes to go see movies with Janet.

☐ The boy went for a walk.
He saw a dog and a bird.
Then it started to rain.

☐ The kids rode their bikes.
Kate's bike is blue and white.
Erin's bike is orange and red.

Key Word Sentences For Note Taking (3) Difficult

☐ Goldilocks sat down in the chair of the great, huge Papa Bear.
It was too hard for her.
Next, she sat in the chair of the Mama Bear .

☐ Cinderella went to the party dressed in a beautiful gown.
She also wore two sparkling glass slippers.
Cinderella knew that when the clock struck midnight, she would have to leave the party.

☐ Snow White wandered through the woods lost and unhappy.
In the clearing she saw a cute little house.
She went up to the front door, and knocked.

☐ The princess remained in the castle for years.
She waited and waited for someone to free her from the witch's evil spell.
But alas, no one came to rescue her.

☐ Once upon a time there were three little pigs.
Each pig wanted to build himself a house.
The first pig met a man selling twigs.

☐ Belle was bored with all the town folk.
She wanted some excitement to come to the town.
The town folk thought that Belle was a little strange.

How To Teach Agents And Their Actions

Prerequisite: Before Agents and Their Actions are taught, the child must understand the concept of All, Some, Never, Few, Many, Most. This is a very advanced activity which the child may or may not be ready for. If the child has difficulty with this drill, the therapist should leave the drill for a considerable amount of time and then revisit it when the child is more able to grasp the abstract concepts which are required for successful completion of this drill.

The therapist should introduce this activity using a very easy animal topic. The therapist should ask the child, "Name some things a dog can do." The therapist should write each suggestion down on the drill sheet. When the child has exhausted his/her suggestions, the therapist should then ask: "Name some things a dog CANNOT do". The child should then suggest things that a dog cannot do. It may be very difficult for the child to associate behaviors that cannot be done by a dog. The therapist should prompt the child if necessary and thereby successfully complete this portion of the drill. Once the list of behaviors that cannot be done has been completed, the therapist should choose the three easiest (most obvious) behaviors that cannot be done and have the child explain why (at the bottom of the sheet). Once the child understands what is required, s/he should be able to do this drill without prompting. Eventually, the child should be able to do this drill completely independently (without the therapist in the room), and without the sheet to use as a visual prompt.

Why Teach Agents and Their Actions?

This drill gives the child the opportunity to describe properties of nouns by what they can and cannot do. In addition, this exercise works on "Why-Because" which is vital to understanding cause and effect, and critical thinking. This drill also works on noun - verb relationships which are important in sentence construction.

Agents and Their Actions

This exercise teaches the child about verbs and verb agents (those who do the action). The child is to name all the different things that an agent can do and a number of things that an agent cannot do. Then the child is asked to answer why the agent cannot do the various things that the child suggests.

Agents and Their Actions

Agent: ____*people*____ (**person**, place, thing)

Things _people_ can do	Things _people_ can't do
work talk smell wink listen hear watch look run walk race ride drive sleep	fly live under water sting (like a bee) go as fast as a car

Questions

WHY CAN'T _people fly_ ? _because they don't have wings._

WHY CAN'T _people live under_ ? _because they don't have gills to breathe with._
water

WHY CAN'T _people sting_ ? _because they don't have a stinger._

How To Teach Verbal Analogies

The therapist introduces this activity by doing a few easy verbal analogies that she knows the child can relate to (such as those on the verbal analogy exercise sheet).

Once the child begins to understand the pattern of this drill, the therapist should fade out the prompts and increase the level of difficulty. The construction of the sentence will most probably need to be "cleaned up" by the therapist until the child understands the way to construct the sentences correctly.

When the child is comfortable with this activity using the sheet, the therapist should remove the sheet and this drill should be done orally with no visual cues.

Why Teach Verbal Analogies?

This drill is designed to concentrate on nouns and the verbs that accompany them. This exercise introduces yet another way to work on the relationship between two parts of language that always go together. The concept of an analogy can be made easy by using extremely obvious analogies about activities that can be observed.

Verbal Analogies

This exercise teaches the concept of an analogy. This is a difficult concept that can be made easy by using extremely obvious analogies about function. Once the child understands these very easy analogies, the analogies can be made less obvious. It is important to remember, however, that most normally developing children do not have a good grasp of abstract analogies.

Verbal Analogies

TYPE: _____Object - action_____

A pencil can write and a knife can cut .

A ball can bounce and a kite can fly .

Scissors can cut and bells can ring .

People talk and birds chirp .

MY OWN ____Object - action____ ANALOGY:

An airplane can fly and a boat can float.

Teaching New Concepts

All the academic concepts included in <u>Teach Me Language</u> have been taught by breaking concepts down into small, manageable segments. It is important to understand how to prepare a concept for instruction because throughout the child's schooling, there will be many new concepts s/he will not pick up through group instruction. The parent or therapist should be kept up-to-date by the school regarding concepts that are difficult for the child. The parent or therapist can teach the child the concept at home to ensure the child will not fall behind the other children. Whenever new concepts need to be taught to the child, the parent or therapist can teach them in the following way:

1. Sequencing Using Visual Representation

For any concept or group of concepts that is ordered (also called a "semantic continuum"), the approach must be to, first, have the child sequence the concept. Sequencing is generally the greatest deficit for children with autism. Before grasping the concept, the child will need to learn how to sequence the concept. Examples of concepts which the child will eventually encounter are: size - small, medium, large; volume - pint, quart, half-gallon (or milliliters); fractions - 1/4, 1/3, 1/2; and continuum concepts such as freezing, cold, warm, hot, boiling.

The therapist should provide a visual representation for each unit or "continuum" concept to be sequenced. The visual representation can be two-dimensional (in the form of pictures or drawings on cards) or three-dimensional (in the form of actual examples of the concept or plastic examples of the concept). The child must be taught to sequence the visual representations of parts of the concept. Once the child can do this, then s/he must learn the written representation of the concept (i.e. the written name). Once the child can use the written representation of the concept, then the child should learn to use the verbal form of the concept.

Note: If the sequence of a concept is too long, the therapist should break it down into 2 or more units first, as was done in this chapter with sequencing money. First the coins were sequenced, and then the bills were sequenced. Finally, both the coins and bills were sequenced together.

2. Comparing Concepts

Once the child can sequence or order the concept, the therapist should have the child compare each concept as it relates to others in its sequence. For example, when sequencing fractions, one is sequencing in terms of size, from smaller portion to larger portion. With time, the feature is amount of time (shorter/longer/more/less time). With semantic word strings like freezing to boiling, the defining feature is temperature (colder/warmer/hotter). The child should be able to answer questions comparing each unit within the concept. S/he will come to understand the concepts if enough time is spent, first using visual representations of the concept, then pairing the words with the visual representations, and finally, providing real-world experience wherever possible.

With Steps 1 and 2, the child should progress from being able to sequence the units of the concepts, to answering the questions 1) with the visual representation, 2) with the written representation only, and 3) with the auditory/verbal representation only (examples of questions include, "Is 1/2 of something larger than 1/3 of something?", or "Is freezing colder than boiling?"). **The goal of all the drills is to reach a point at which the child does not rely on visual cues or representations, but uses his/her listening skills to comprehend and communicate. This point cannot be overemphasized!**

3. Teaching equivalent units/sets

Whenever possible, the therapist should first teach the concept visually using a matching task. Some concepts will be easier to do this with than others. Fractions are easy to match since two 1/4 fractional parts match one 1/2 fractional part, etc. With ordered concepts ("semantic continuum" concepts), the therapist must teach equivalent words or synonyms whenever possible. For example, freezing can be represented by a picture and by the synonym "very cold".

Note: These steps are not comprehensive because each concept has unique properties that will call for customization. The above directions are a guide to focus the teaching which will make the concept being taught clearer for the child. Through all of the material that the therapist introduces, there are recurring concepts that the child may have difficulty with. Examples of these recurring concepts are "enough, not enough" and "same/alike/both, different/not the same." These recurring concepts should be taught and focused upon at all times.

The following is a partial list of concepts that can, eventually, be approached using the above technique:

money	family trees
time	history
sizes	time lines
temperature	age
weights	measures of sound
fractions	ordinal position
units of measurement	place value
geometry	

These concepts should NOT be introduced all at once! It is important to have no more than two concepts introduced at the same time. Some children will require that only one concept be introduced at any one time; other children will be able to handle two concepts in the same session. If too many concepts are introduced at once, the child may confuse the "defining features" of each concept. The more similar concepts the child grasps, the easier it will be for the child to learn other concepts. For example, once the child understands time concepts well, money concepts should be easier for him/her to learn.

Why Must Concepts Be Taught This Way?

Most children with pervasive developmental disorders learn better through visual and "hands on" representation of concepts, as opposed to when they are presented orally. Therefore, if one teaches the concept using a visual representation, it will be easier for the child to grasp. It is important to pair the visual representation with words so that the child understands the concept when it is used or referred to verbally. Sequencing is at the heart of most difficult concepts for the child; therefore, by teaching concepts as described above, the sequencing problem is attacked directly.

7 Therapy Schedules

Setting Up a Therapy Schedule
- Start with the Easiest Drills First
- Customize to the Individual Child
- Drills Given Are Simply an Arsenal

Simplified Schedule For The Child

Independent Work Instrument

Beginning Schedule - Level 1

Beginning Schedule - Level 2

Intermediate Schedule

Advanced Schedule

Setting Up A Therapy Schedule

This chapter is designed to give guidelines to setting up a language therapy program. It is important, however, to understand that these are just guidelines since every child differs in level of ability and amount of time that s/he is able to sit with a therapist and do these activities. Clearly, younger children should not be required to sit as long as older children without breaks; however, some young children enjoy doing these types of activities and are prepared to sit for longer periods of time. The ideal scenario is to have the child work two hours a day on these activities; however, less time is still adequate. It is important to understand, however, that a child who is worked with minimally i.e. once a week, will not progress very quickly, and in some cases will not be able to grasp some of the more difficult, but necessary, concepts. The following guidelines are:

① Start with the Easiest Drills First

It is better to start with drills that the child is certain to understand even if those drills are too easy for the child. In this way, the child will feel good about the therapy and eventually the therapist will come to understand the appropriate level for that child. If the parent is to be working with the child, this guideline is extremely important since parents often assume that their child is more advanced than is the case and begin at too high a level.

② Customize to the Individual Child

Every drill in this book is given in a generic form to apply to as many situations as possible. This is why it is very important to customize each drill to the individual child. For example, if the child likes Kentucky Fried Chicken instead of McDonald's, use KFC in the drill instead of McDonalds.

Customization is also important in terms of the therapy schedules that have been provided. These are only suggestions of how to start a language therapy program. If the child can do more drills than we have suggested in the beginning therapy schedule, it is fine to add a few more drills (keeping in mind guideline 1. above). In addition, the therapy schedules given for the advanced student should be modified to keep up with the child's ability. Once the child has firmly internalized a concept, MOVE ON!

③ Drills Given Are Simply an Arsenal

The drills described in this book all attempt to attack language deficits in a unique way. If one drill is not making sense to the child, it is important to look for another drill that will work on the same problem in a different way. Once the reader understands the way these children think and assimilate knowledge and concepts, s/he will be able to create drills which follow the same pattern.

Simplified Schedule For The Child

This is a sample of a therapy schedule that the child can relate to. In this way, the child see what is on the agenda and knows that in order to receive the reward at the bottom of the page, s/he must go through the schedule. The treat at the bottom should be something the child chooses (within reason) so that the child is motivated.

Today's Work Schedule

1 Read about _____ Frogs _____

2 Make an outline and talk about _____ Frogs _____

3 Write a story _____ Two girls at the park _____

4 Answer questions _____ about calendar _____

5 ___ Do reading comprehension _____

6 Talk about what I did today

7 Practice talking and having a conversation

8 ___ Do math problems _____

9 Work by myself: do independent work

When I am done, I get to: _____ eat a cupcake _____

Independent Work Instrument

This sheet is designed to teach the child to do his/her work independently. This is also a good check as to whether the child is becoming too dependent on the therapist to complete his/her work. The items to put on the independent work sheet are drills that the child has mastered and can do ALONE without any help. The therapist should NOT have the child work on difficult activities independently since this will create frustration rather than a sense of accomplishment.

Independent Work

Check off each square when you are done.

☐ math word problems

☐ word pairs

☐ brainstorming

☐ writing a story

Let me know when you are done.

Beginning Schedule - Level 1

This weekly schedule is designed for the therapy manager to monitor how often various activities are being done. This is the beginning level in which the following drills are recommended. This is, however, only a suggestion since every child is different. Therapist should check the schedule before starting the therapy session each day and begin with the drills that were not done during the last therapy session.

Level 1 Weekly Drill/Activity Record Week Of: _____								
Goal Areas	**How Often**	S	M	T	W	TH	F	S
Reading - Stories								
Reading - Topic Based								
Animal (1 per week))								
Animal Outline								
Language								
Structured Story Pre-Writing	Daily							
Critical Thinking								
Emotions (1 every week or two)	Daily							
1 Sequence (from a daily routine)								
Contingent Words								
Word Associations								
Conversation								
Reciprocal Comments	Daily							
Answering Topic Based Questions	Daily							

Record the factual reading drills from Chapter 3 in this area ➡

Record the various language drills (in this case from Chapter 5 in this area ➡

Record the critical thinking and logic drills in this area ➡

Record the social conversation drills in this area ➡

Notes: _____

_____

_____

Beginning Schedule - Level 2

This weekly schedule is designed for the therapy manager to monitor how often various activities are being done. This is the beginning level in which the following drills are recommended. This is, however, only a suggestion since every child is different.

Record the reading comprehension drills from Chapter 6 in this area ➤

Record the factual reading drills from Chapter 3 in this area ➤

Record the various language drills (in this case from Chapter 5 in this area ➤

Record the critical thinking and logic drills in this area ➤

Record the social conversation drills in this area ➤

Level 2 Weekly Drill/Activity Record

Week Of: _____

Goal Areas	How Often	S	M	T	W	TH	F	S
Reading - Stories								
Begin Reading Comprehension	Daily							
Reading - Topic Based								
Animal (1 per week))								
Animal Outline								
Animal Definitions								
Animal Mixed Questions								
Language								
Structured Story Pre-Writing	Daily							
Critical Thinking								
Emotions (1 every week or two) Daily								
1 Sequence (from a daily routine)								
Contingent Words								
Word Associations								
Conversation								
Recall of Day	Daily							
Reciprocal Comments	Daily							
Answering Simple Word Questions	Daily							
Finding Out About Someone	Daily							

Notes: _____

_____

_____

Intermediate Schedule

This weekly schedule is designed for the therapy manager to monitor how often various activities are being done. This is the beginning level in which the following drills are recommended. This is, however, only a suggestion since every child is different.

Intermediate Weekly Drill/Activity Record

Week Of: _____

Goal Areas	How Often	S	M	T	W	TH	F	S
Reading - Stories								
Reading Comp. (1 per week, daily review)								
Reading - Topic Based								
Animal maintenance (Grids)								
Occupations (1 per week, daily review)								
Occupation Outline								
Occupation Mixed Questions								
Language								
Structured Story Pre-Writing	Daily							
Structured Story Writing	Daily							
Answering Math Word Problems								
True or False Questions	Daily							
Making Comparisons	Daily							
Critical Thinking								
Safe/Dangerous Script	Daily							
Contingent Words								
Emotions - cause/effect								
Sequencing (simple numerical & situational)								
Conversation								
Recall of Day	Daily							
Reciprocal Comments	Daily							
Answering Topic Based Questions	Daily							
Finding Out About Someone	Daily							

Record the reading comprehension drills from Chapter 6 in this area ⟶

Record the factual reading drills from Chapter 3 in this area ⟶

Record the various language drills in this area ⟶

Record the critical thinking and logic drills in this area ⟶

Record the social conversation drills in this area ⟶

Notes: _____
_____
_____

Advanced Schedule

This weekly schedule is designed for the therapy manager to monitor how often various activities are being done. This is the beginning level in which the following drills are recommended. This is, however, only a suggestion since every child is different.

Record the reading comprehension drills from Chapter 6 in this area ➡

Record the factual reading drills from Chapter 3 in this area ➡

Record the various language drills (in this case from Chapter 5 in this area ➡

Record the critical thinking and logic drills in this area ➡

Record the social conversation drills in this area ➡

Advanced Weekly Drill/Activity Record

Week Of: _____

Goal Areas	How Often	S	M	T	W	TH	F	S
Reading - Stories								
Reading Comp (1 per week, daily review)								
Reading - Topic Based								
Occupations (1 per week, daily review)								
Occupation Outline								
Mixed Questions								
Language								
Wh & True or False Questions	Daily							
Comparisons	Daily							
Vocabulary	3 x a week							
Time Concepts	Daily							
Math Word Problems (creating/constraining)								
Key word note-taking/listening	Daily							
Writing Stories & Pre-Writing	Daily							
Critical Thinking								
Safe/Dangerous Script	Daily							
Identifying Safe/Dangerous	Daily							
Problem/Solution Script	Daily							
Identifying Problem/Solution	Daily							
Verbal Problem/Solution	Daily							
Emotions -cause/effect	Daily							
Sequencing								
Conversation								
Recall of Day	Daily							
Reciprocal Comments	Daily							
Answering Topic Based Questions	Daily							
Finding Out About Someone	Daily							

Notes: _____

_____

_____

Index

O

object functions 2, 254
occupations 2, 104, 125, 128, 129, 140, 142-144, 147, 155, 158-159, 185, 192, 403-404
opinions 16, 30, 32, 90-92, 94-101
oral definitions 2, 107-108, 121, 129-130, 140, 146, 149, 153
oral/written definitions 2, 104
orally defining words 2, 254
ordering information 2, 254
ordering my food 2, 16
outline 399, 401-404
outline for topical information 2, 108, 114-117, 129, 133-136, 146, 149

P

paragraph writing 2, 170, 216, 231-235, 245
pervasive developmental disorders 2, 6-8
phonics 7
phrase identification 170, 207
place value 2, 254
planets 2, 104, 105, 153, 154
pre-story writing 2, 170, 401-404
prepositions 2, 6, 8, 213
pretend play 2, 16, 23-24
problems 2, 9, 11-12, 16, 23, 29, 42, 62, 66-70, 72-74, 76-77, 79-81, 104, 120, 122, 139, 141
problems and solutions 2, 16, 404
professions 4, 104-105, 128-130, 132, 137-139, 141, 143, 146, 153
profession fill-in the blanks 2, 104
pronouns 170-174, 212
proud 2, 16, 55, 60

Q

questions 2, 6, 11, 16, 106-107, 109, 120, 124-125, 128, 139, 144, 166

R

reading 2, 6-9, 105-107, 111-112, 118, 128, 137, 146
Reading - Stories 401-404
Reading - Topic Based 401-404
reading comprehension 2, 170, 254, 265-275, 277-278, 283, 298, 399, 402-404
recall 2, 10-11, 112, 170
recall of day 402-404
recall of significant daily events 217, 250
reciprocal comments 2, 16, 42, 401, 402, 403, 404
repetition 2, 4, 8, 104
reptiles 108, 110, 119
rules for talking with friends 2, 16, 31

S

sad 2, 16, 55, 57, 59, 62-66, 72, 74, 82-83, 98
safe 11
safe and dangerous 2, 16, 67, 69, 71-72, 403-404
scared 2, 16, 55, 59
schedule 2-4, 10, 12, 398-404